Praise for REAL SUPERFOO

"It's amazing how fulfilling it can be to give your body the optimal fuel.
Ocean Robbins will show you how to take delicious action—so you can enjoy
a clearer mind, a healthier body, and a more satisfying life."

— **Tony Robbins**, #1 *New York Times* best-selling author and peak performance strategist

"The best superfoods are loaded with antioxidants and other phytonutrients that can help
you to lose weight, lower your blood pressure, live longer, and feel better. *Real Superfoods*
illuminates the proven benefits of some of the most truly 'super' foods in the world."

— **Michael Greger, M.D.**, best-selling author of *How Not to Die*
and founder of NutritionFacts.org

"A must-have cookbook for anyone looking to optimize their health and well-being.
It cuts through conflicting and confusing nutritional advice and offers a practical path to
slow the aging process through ordinary, easily accessible, and inexpensive ingredients."

— **Mark Hyman, M.D.**, best-selling author and founder
and director of The UltraWellness Center

"Good news! The healthiest superfoods can also be the most delicious and affordable.
And what's good for you is also good for our planet. In this extraordinary book,
Ocean and Nichole show us how and why. Highly recommended!"

— **Dean Ornish, M.D.**, #1 *New York Times* best-selling author
and founder of the Preventive Medicine Research Institute

"It is pure culinary genius—creative, innovative, and absolutely
brimming with wise and wonderful insights."

— **Brenda Davis, R.D.**, author of *Becoming Vegan* and plant-based pioneer

"Empowers you to maximize nutrition on any budget and, with its delicious recipes,
helps you create delicious dishes that everyone will love. Get this book and start cookin'!"

— **Michael Klaper, M.D.**, director of the Moving Medicine Forward initiative

"Ocean Robbins brilliantly demystifies nutritious eating in *Real Superfoods*. A must-read
for anyone seeking improved health through everyday plant-based foods."

— **Dr. Will Bulsiewicz**, *New York Times* best-selling author of *The Fiber Fueled Cookbook*

"A friendly and practical road map to greater health, vitality, and comfort in the kitchen. This book is a joy to read—and the recipes are wholesome, affordable, and delectable."

— **Susan Peirce Thompson, Ph.D.**, professor and *New York Times* best-selling author of *Bright Line Eating*

"An extraordinary and powerful guide to the care and nourishment of the human body. It provides insightful and common-sense recommendations that can help anyone achieve optimal health and well-being."

— **Drs. Dean and Ayesha Sherzai,** neuroscientists and best-selling authors of *The Alzheimer's Solution*

"The wisdom in this beautiful book is simple and yet utterly profound. The research is on point, and the recipes are amazing. Do yourself— and your microbiome—a huge favor: read *Real Superfoods* today!"

— **Robynne Chutkan, M.D.,** author of *Gutbliss, The Microbiome Solution*, and *The Anti-Viral Gut*

"Introduces the amazing benefits of some of the most potent health-boosting foods on the planet—and shows you how to make them super delicious."

— **Thom Hartmann,** talk show host and *New York Times* best-selling author

REAL
SUPERFOODS

Also by Ocean Robbins

31-Day Food Revolution: Heal Your Body, Feel Great, and Transform Your World

Voices of the Food Revolution: You Can Heal Your Body and Your World—with Food!

The Power of Partnership: Building Healing Bridges Across Historic Divides

Choices for Our Future: A Generation Rising for Life on Earth

Also by Nichole Dandrea-Russert, MS, RDN

The Fiber Effect: Stop Counting Calories and Start Counting Fiber for Better Health

The Vegan Athlete's Nutrition Handbook: The Essential Guide for Plant-Based Performance

REAL SUPERFOODS

EVERYDAY INGREDIENTS TO ELEVATE YOUR HEALTH

OCEAN ROBBINS

AND NICHOLE DANDREA-RUSSERT, MS, RDN

HAY HOUSE LLC

Carlsbad, California • New York City

London • Sydney • New Delhi

Copyright © 2023 by Food Revolution Network

Published in the United States by: Hay House LLC: www.hayhouse.com®
Published in Australia by: Hay House Australia Publishing Pty Ltd: www.hayhouse.com.au
Published in the United Kingdom by: Hay House UK Ltd: www.hayhouse.co.uk
Published in India by: Hay House Publishers (India) Pty Ltd: www.hayhouse.co.in

Indexer: Jay Kreider
Cover design: The Book Designers
Interior design: Michelle Farinella
Photography: Angela MacNeil Photography

All rights reserved. No part of this book may be reproduced by any mechanical, photographic, or electronic process, or in the form of a phonographic recording; nor may it be stored in a retrieval system, transmitted, or otherwise be copied for public or private use—other than for "fair use" as brief quotations embodied in articles and reviews—without prior written permission of the publisher.

The author of this book does not dispense medical advice or prescribe the use of any technique as a form of treatment for physical, emotional, or medical problems without the advice of a physician, either directly or indirectly. The intent of the author is only to offer information of a general nature to help you in your quest for emotional, physical, and spiritual well-being. In the event you use any of the information in this book for yourself, the author and the publisher assume no responsibility for your actions.

Library of Congress Cataloging-in-Publication Data
Names: Robbins, Ocean, 1973- author. | Dandrea-Russert, Nichole, author.
Title: Real superfoods : everyday ingredients to elevate your health /
  Ocean Robbins, Nichole Dandrea-Russert, RDN.
Description: 1st edition. | Carlsbad, California : Hay House, Inc., [2023]
Identifiers: LCCN 2023026139 | ISBN 9781401973360 (hardback) | ISBN
  9781401973377 (ebook)
Subjects: LCSH: Cooking (Natural foods) | Nutrition. | LCGFT: Cookbooks.
Classification: LCC TX741 .R5924 2023 | DDC 641.5/637--dc23/eng/20230616
LC record available at https://lccn.loc.gov/2023026139

Tradepaper ISBN: 978-1-4019-9322-1
E-book ISBN: 978-1-4019-7337-7
Audiobook ISBN: 978-1-4019-7338-4

10 9 8 7 6 5 4 3 2 1
1st edition, October 2023
2nd edition, January 2025

Printed in China

This product uses responsibly sourced papers and/or recycled materials. For more information, see www.hayhouse.com.

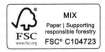

To you, dear reader, may this book inspire you to add more plants to your plate; spark creativity in your kitchen; and spread plant-based goodness to your family, friends, and community.

Cheers to good health for you and the planet.

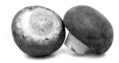

CONTENTS

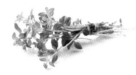

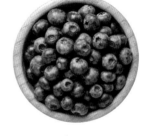

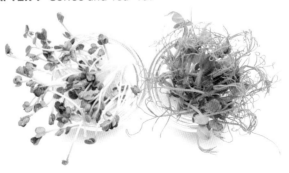

PART TWO: REAL SUPERFOODS RECIPES

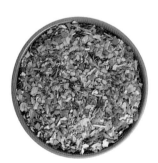

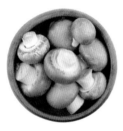

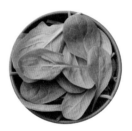

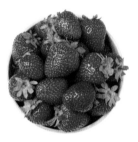

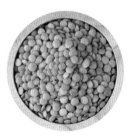

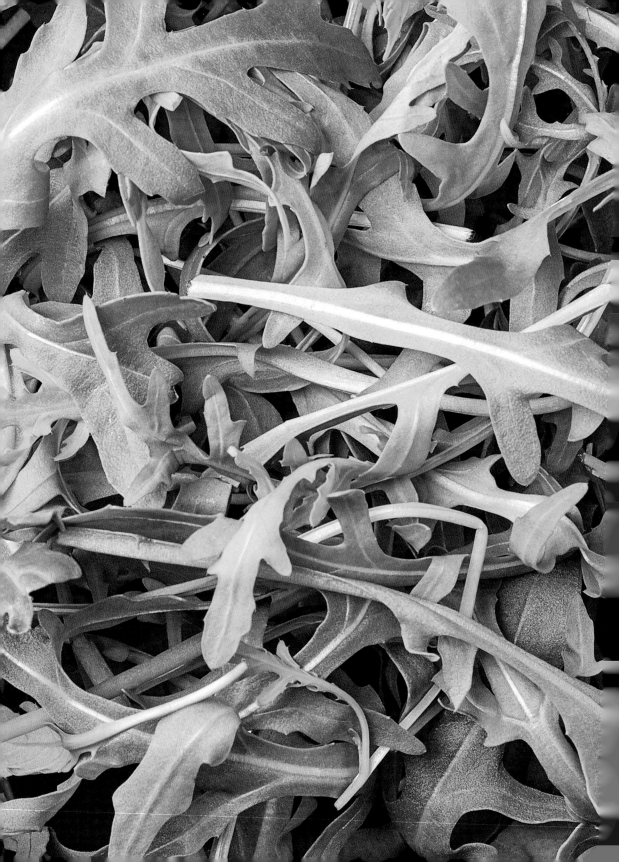

FOREWORD
BY HAILE THOMAS

As a speaker, wellness and compassion activist, and writer, I've found storytelling to be one of the most potent tools to prompt connection and transformation. It provides space for our wholeness—the entirety of our experiences—to be recognized so we may find new, softer ways to grow. Our stories comprise many dimensions, and food is one of them. I would know! My very own journey into food and nutrition began with my family's successful reversal of my dad's type-2 diabetes without the use of medication (thanks to the adoption of a primarily plant-based diet), inspiring over a decade of local and global work to bring wellness education and empowerment to my Gen Z peers.

Food is our origin, the source of our bodily maintenance, a tool for nurturing our potential, and a medium through which we learn about and explore our cultural roots, as well as our expanding and intersecting worlds. We are intricately connected to one another—to life—through food. Ocean's story, wisdom, and continued service to hundreds of thousands of people through the mission of delivering healthy, ethical, and sustainable food for all at the Food Revolution Network beautifully illuminates this interconnectivity. He is a food advocate and educator I trust and deeply admire. Ocean's dedication and pursuits are shining examples of the community we find when we commune with nature and lean in to the nourishment offered.

By helping bring my dad into good health all those years ago, I was introduced to the abundance of healing properties in veggies, like antioxidant-filled leafy greens and protein-packed legumes. And in striking contrast, I also discovered the horrors of a food industry that profits by exploiting something so precious and essential to life: health. And not just the health of people like you and me but that of land animals and sea

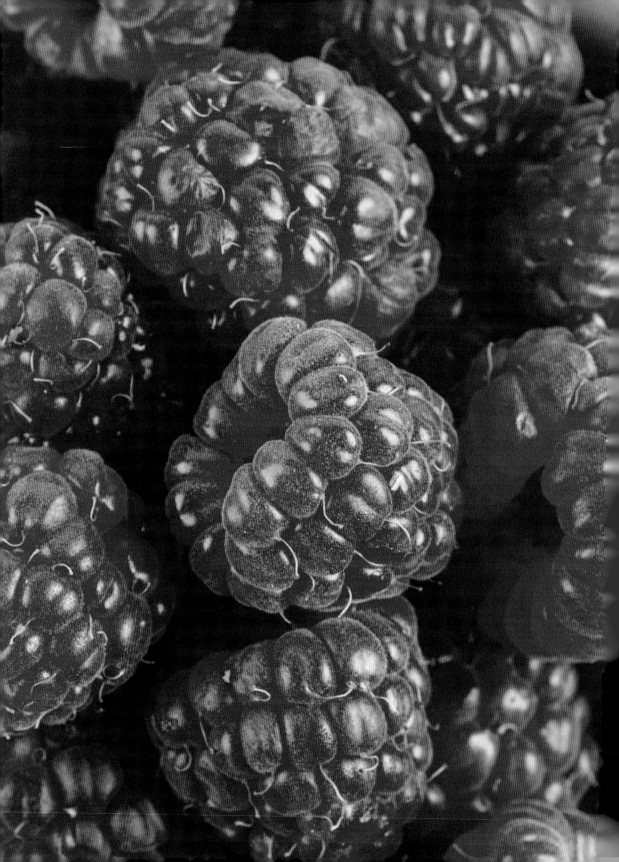

creatures, and the forests, bodies of water, and airways that maintain our ecosystems. These life-giving sources are relentlessly desecrated by the mass impact of unsustainable, inhumane, cheap, low-quality food production. Like mirrors to each other, Earth and an extensive global population are suffering from symptoms of neglect, appearing in the form of chronic illnesses directly connected to diet and lifestyle choices.

Thankfully *Real Superfoods* offers a shining path forward in the face of this dark reality, starting with what's on our plates. Through scientific evidence of the incredible benefits of plant foods, delectable and simple recipes ready for your creative input or cultural twists, and stories of the great joy and good health brought about by our plant friends, we see a new vision emerging—a vision of allyship and care between humans, plants, and all living beings.

Nature is in service to all parts of itself—us included—and this network of support can inspire us to live life with greater purpose, intentionality, and community care.

We can't do life alone. And thanks to the expertise and insight of Ocean and Nichole, *Real Superfoods* offers a (cruciferous or maybe tuberous) hand to hold as we journey on, with digestible and practical guidance to fuel our road ahead.

Real Superfoods prompts us to edit the narratives (and systems) that have created exclusionary perceptions of highly nutritious foods, resulting in limited access to certain groups of people. And by incorporating more "everyday" plant foods into our diets, preserving our personal health transforms into advocacy for a better, healthier world at large, where thriving is defined by feeling good and not the facades we've been fed.

— **Haile Thomas**
Author of *Living Lively* and co-founder of Matcha Thomas

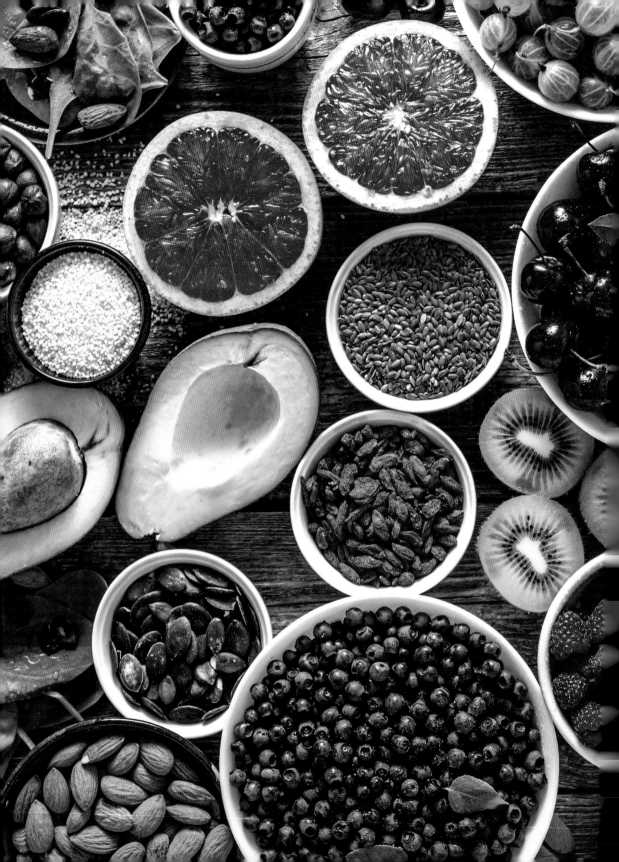

INTRODUCTION

Let's start this book with a story.

My grandfather Irvine (Irv) Robbins and great-uncle Burt (Butch) Baskin founded the Baskin-Robbins ice cream company in 1945. Through clever marketing (31-derful flavors, one for every day of the month) and a then-novel business model (franchising), they grew the company into a huge American success story. My dad, John Robbins, Grandpa Irv's only son, grew up swimming in an ice cream cone–shaped swimming pool, eating enormous amounts of ice cream, and inventing new flavors. Everyone, especially Grandpa Irv, expected him to follow in the footsteps of his wildly successful father and take over the family business once he became an adult.

Imagine my grandpa's shock and disappointment when my dad, along with his bride (my mom-to-be), Deo, walked away from the business and the wealth it represented to live a simpler life in harmony with nature and all life-forms. They moved to a tiny island off the coast of British Columbia, where they built a one-room log cabin, grew most of their own food, practiced yoga and meditation for several hours each day, and lived on less than $1,000 a year.

That's where I was born. Whether I grew up extremely poor or immeasurably rich is a matter of perspective.

From my grandparents' perspective, I was practically starving. No ice cream, no steak, no fast food, and no candy. My dad had renounced any access to or dependence on the family wealth, in addition to any leadership of Baskin-Robbins.

From my parents' perspective, we were thriving. We grew much of our food and supplemented with the least expensive natural staples available. Every fall, we'd get a delivery of 25-pound sacks of dried legumes and grains, cases of potatoes and winter squash, a year's supply of herbs and spices, and some fresh fruits and vegetables. We'd go through the produce quickly, before it spoiled, and portion out the rest to last us until the following spring, when our garden would take up the slack. And we had Siberian kale growing in our garden all winter; we just brushed off the snow and it was fabulous.

My dad's family of origin enjoyed a diet that many people around the world aspire to. It included meals at fine restaurants and plenty of steaks, processed foods, rich desserts, and of course, lots and lots of ice cream. This diet was rich in calories but lacking in nutrients. And over time, the huge quantities of sugar, saturated fat, salt, highly processed grains, and artificial ingredients began to wreak havoc on their health. My great-uncle Burt Baskin was the first to fall, dying of a heart attack at the age of 54.

My dad's uncle was one of the most successful entrepreneurs in American history. He had a family he loved and work he enjoyed. But he didn't have his health, and he left my great-aunt Shirley a widow and his kids (my dad's cousins) fatherless.

My folks and I, on the other hand, ate an entirely whole foods, plant-based diet. No refined sugar, no white flour, no preservatives or additives, and no meat or dairy. I grew up strong and healthy on this diet; in elementary school I set pull-up and push-up records, and I completed my first marathon when I was 10. My parents likewise enjoyed rich health, as my mom became a dance workshop leader, and my dad went on to coach a track team and to become a triathlete.

When it comes to food, most people think that they have to choose between good-tasting and "good for you." American wit and drama critic Alexander Woollcott spoke for many when he complained, "Everything I like is either illegal, immoral, or fattening."

And my family's story could appear to reinforce that forced choice. Our relatives believed we had given up earthly pleasures in exchange for puritanical misery. Sure, we might live longer, but at the cost of renouncing everything that made life worth living. What was the point?

What they didn't know was how delicious healthy food can taste when you give your taste buds a break from hyperpalatable processed foods and animal products. What they never experienced was the wonderful feeling of being nourished, rather than punished, by their diet. What they missed was the mental clarity and physical vigor that can accompany a simple lifestyle in tune with nature.

And they also missed some really good recipes—which prove that when you know what to do with wholesome ingredients, you can make them taste amazing.

The way we ate, and the way we still eat, is a win-win: pleasure in the short term and well-being in the longer term. I wrote this book (to complement the amazing recipes from Nichole Dandrea-Russert, RDN), so you can experience a similar win-win in your life and have the tools and confidence to share it with loved ones. I want you to try a few recipes, to discover that healthy food can be twice as pleasurable as the standard modern diet. First, you'll love these foods when you eat them. Then, you'll love how you feel later: minutes later, hours later, and years later.

Foods and Superfoods

One of the most common criticisms of the whole foods, plant-based diet is that it's elitist: too expensive for ordinary people to afford and too alien to their traditional palates. My family's experience proves that this doesn't have to be the case. Yet there's some truth to the elitist argument.

Part of the reason healthy food can be more expensive than unhealthy food is structural; various governmental subsidies make sugar, corn syrup, factory-farmed meat and dairy, white flour, and low-quality oils much cheaper to consumers than their true costs. For people of extremely limited means, the cheapest calories in the grocery store are found in the snack aisle rather than the produce section. Also, many marginalized communities are "food deserts," where it can be easier to access fried pork rinds than a fresh tomato.

But a big reason many people think healthy food is expensive is the ever-expanding marketing efforts from the

health food and wellness industries. In addition to the billions of dollars spent annually on supplements, consumers have, in recent decades, been enticed to purchase expensive "functional" foods to boost their immune systems, balance their nervous systems, and avoid disease, disability, and premature death.

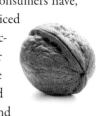

To promote this spending, marketers invented a new category: superfoods.

When we hear the word *superfood*, most of us think of the fruits, roots, or leaves of species found only in faraway, inaccessible places: high in the Himalayas (goji berries) or deep in the Amazon basin (acai berries). We're told that they're exceptionally high in powerful nutrients such as antioxidants and adaptogens.

In fact, *superfood* is a marketing term rather than an accurate assessment of nutritional value. If it were about nutrition alone, we would expect to see the wellness industry promote the same superfoods year after year. Instead, hot new superfoods hit the shelves all the time. They show up in powdered supplements or in trendy dishes like acai bowls. Your local natural foods store and the nearby upscale supermarket chain likely advertise these products in commercials and weekly fliers.

And the main reason they attract such big advertising budgets? Profit margin.

If a company can mark up a product a lot—and especially if that product is nonperishable—they have incentive to invest in marketing it and bringing ever more of the "superfood" to the world.

I'm not saying these products lack nutritional value; many of them may very well perform as promised. But however high they are in antioxidants and other nutrients of interest, they're just as high— or higher—in price. In fact, many are simply too expensive for the average person.

Ginseng, for example, can cost $1 per gram or more. That's around 50 times higher than a super-healthy commonplace spice like oregano, which you can buy for around 2 cents per gram.

The high prices of exotically sourced superfoods may reflect their scarcity, the labor that goes into growing and harvesting them, and the overhead gleaned by distributors and marketers who see the potential for huge financial returns. And in terms of environmental costs, they often leave a higher carbon footprint than locally sourced foods and ingredients.

No doubt many of these foods are potent, but how "super" is a food that only the wealthiest can afford? Superheroes don't just save rich clients from collapsing buildings and train tracks—they exist to do good for as many people as possible. We want our superfoods to be nutrient dense to be sure, brimming with antioxidants, flavonoids, and other potent and beneficial micronutrients. But we also want them to be affordable and accessible.

Also, true superheroes don't harm one group to save another. Superman never tore the beam from one building to reinforce a different one. Unfortunately, the global popularity of expensive superfoods can actually harm the local communities who've been tending, harvesting, and benefiting from them for millennia. As global demand for an exotic superfood increases, so too does its price. Indigenous communities who may rely upon them for their own nutritional needs find themselves "outbid" by wealthier foreigners. And increased demand can lead to land use change and water depletion, damaging those indigenous ecosystems.

So the mission of this book is to introduce you to superfoods that check all the boxes. They're nutritional powerhouses that can enhance your health and vitality. They're affordable and easily accessible supermarket foods. And when you know what to do with them, they can be super delicious, too! You're probably familiar with all of them but haven't realized how fabulous they are—or could be—with the help of a great recipe.

Where Is the Real Treasure?

An old Hasidic folk tale tells of Eizek, a man from the city of Krakow who dreams of a treasure hidden under a bridge in Prague, 300 miles away. After having the same dream each night for a week, he decides to undertake the long and arduous journey to dig up and claim the treasure. When he arrives, however, he finds a platoon of soldiers guarding the bridge night and day. There is no way he can dig without arousing their attention and ire.

After wandering around the bridge for a few days, Eizek is confronted by a soldier: "What are you doing here?" Flustered, he blurts out the truth about his dream. The soldier laughs in derision and says, "Are you so naive to believe in dreams? I keep having a dream that if I travel to Krakow and dig underneath the house of a man named Eizek, I shall find a treasure. Do you think I'm going to travel 300 miles just because of a silly dream?"

Stunned, Eizek returns home, gets a shovel, and discovers a treasure buried under his own house.

Modern wellness seekers are a bit like Eizek. We've been told repeatedly that the elixirs of life can be found only on the other side of the world, and we must pay dearly for access to them.

And like Eizek, after scouring the globe for the most fantastic health-promoting, longevity-bestowing, vigor-imparting foods, we learn that we've had treasures in our own backyard all along. Treasures that we've overlooked or taken for granted, like leafy greens, mushrooms, lentils and beans, berries, onions and garlic, herbs and spices, sweet potatoes, nuts and seeds, and coffee and tea. Ordinary, everyday fare that in many cases is even more nutrient rich than the heavily marketed superfoods from distant locales.

What's at Stake

Let's not sugarcoat it: the modern diet is a nutritional and environmental disaster.

Nutritionally, we are calorie rich and nutrient poor, overdosing daily on harmful and inflammatory foods. Being overweight or obese are among the leading indicators of this situation, showing up long before most people develop one or more of the chronic diseases that also result from the typical modern diet.

In the US, roughly 42 percent of adults are clinically obese, up from 30 percent in 1999.[1]

Among the possible outcomes of obesity are a higher risk of developing serious diseases and conditions, including heart disease, stroke, type 2 diabetes, and certain types of cancer. And these are all among the top 10 leading causes of death in the US,[2] to say nothing of the pain, suffering, and disability that accompany them.

Other conditions strongly linked to diet include Alzheimer's, gallbladder disease, arthritis, sleep apnea, asthma, reproductive issues, autoimmune diseases, digestive problems, depression, and anxiety.[3] And one of the main organs of protection in our bodies, the microbiome, grows ever weaker as plummeting diversity of beneficial bacteria further compromises our immune, digestive, cognitive, and mental health.

The modern diet doesn't just harm the individuals who consume it and those who must take care of them. It's also a leading contributor to public health catastrophes that can affect us all. Due in part to the huge quantities of antibiotics added to livestock feed, antibiotic-resistant bacteria have emerged that undermine our ability to treat infectious diseases. It's not just overzealous doctors overprescribing amoxicillin for every earache or sore throat. In some countries, up to 80 percent of the medically important antibiotics in circulation[4] are given to livestock at "subtherapeutic" doses; that is, they don't treat already-sick animals

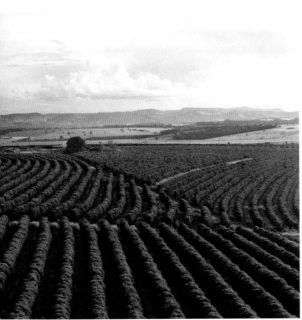

but instead serve to keep herds and flocks from developing illnesses while they live in conditions of overcrowding and filth.

Beyond the immeasurable cost in terms of physical and emotional suffering, the epidemics of chronic disease are also undermining the economy. The economic burden of Alzheimer's disease in the US alone was estimated to approach $305 billion in 2020, including the costs of productivity loss, health care and skilled care, and the sacrifices made by family members and friends to provide informal care to those afflicted. Demographers point out that in the next generation, that number is likely to triple.[5]

And Alzheimer's is just the tip of the iceberg when it comes to the financial burden of dealing with all this chronic disease. As far back as 2004, General Motors estimated that the cost of providing health care to its employees added an average of $1,200 to the price of every car it sold—more even than the cost of the steel used to make the vehicle.[6] In fact, in 2020, what we call "health care" (I think it would be more accurate to call it "disease symptom management") absorbed nearly 20 percent of the entirety of the US gross domestic product—more than four times the amount of money spent on the world's largest military budget.[7, 8]

And that's just the human-centric view. When you look at the planet itself, the problem grows even more dire. Industrial agriculture is one of the world's largest contributors to greenhouse gas emissions. The destruction of rainforests in favor of cattle grazing or for land on which to grow soy (mostly to feed to livestock), as well as the destruction of peat bogs for palm oil plantations, are eliminating two of the main ways the earth stores carbon. Increasing carbon in the atmosphere has already destabilized the world's weather patterns, making dry places dryer and wet places wetter, raising sea levels, and leading to more frequent catastrophic crop failures.

We're draining our aquifers in order to irrigate land for livestock feed, and returning some of the water—now polluted with animal waste—to our lakes, rivers, and groundwater.

All this environmental destruction might seem easier to justify if it was somehow essential to feeding humanity. But it's not.

In a world in which hundreds of millions of people struggle with hunger and food insecurity, animal agriculture is actually part of the problem.

That's because meat production turns out to be profoundly inefficient. Animals are the proverbial middlemen (or middle-cows, as the case may sometimes be) in the system. Globally, livestock provides just 18 percent of calories but takes up 83 percent of all global farmland.[9]

How wasteful is that? The most efficient meat, chicken, requires an estimated nine calories of feed to create a single calorie of edible chicken. Bruce Friedrich, executive director at the Good Food Institute, likens this to making nine plates of pasta and tossing eight of them in the trash.[10] According to Friedrich, the ratio for pork is 15 to 1, which still looks good compared to the most inefficient meat of all: beef, which needs 25 calories of feed to produce one beef calorie.

Every calorie of feed produces a relatively small amount of meat, eggs, or dairy products. The rest is turned into hooves, hides, bones, feathers, body heat, energy to move the animals around, and, of course, manure.

Livestock production is basically a protein factory in reverse.

That wastefulness might be fine if all people in the world were adequately fed. But according to recent reports, over 800 million people are chronically hungry.[11] Not only do they struggle to afford meat, but many of them have also lost the ability to grow their own food due to the land use demands of animal agriculture. We can feed the whole world; we just can't do it with meat.

Why Real Superfoods?
(aka "The Good News")

Our mission at Food Revolution Network is "healthy, ethical, and sustainable food for all." Food that's healthy nourishes our bodies rather than causing them harm. Food that's ethical makes life better for everyone rather than causing some to suffer so that others may be well fed. And food that's sustainable honors the living planet upon which it grows, rather than destroying the environment to increase short-term profitability.

Exotic and expensive superfoods can't provide healthy, ethical, and sustainable food for all. Instead, we need superfoods that are super for your health, super for your wallet, and super for the earth.

Writer and food activist Michael Pollan's seven-word phrase pretty much sums up our philosophy: "Eat food. Not too much. Mostly plants." (By "food," he means real food that our great-grandparents would have recognized, as opposed to the food-like products manufactured out of highly processed and artificial ingredients.)

If you have the resources, you can also go the extra step of voting with your dollars for local, organic, and fair-trade foods when possible. Doing so will benefit your health, the well-being of the workers and communities where the food is produced, and the planet as a whole.

So that's the good news: you can start making a positive difference for the future of life on Earth with your next meal. You can vote with your dollars for a more ethical and sustainable food system. You can choose foods with a low carbon and water footprint. You can opt for food that doesn't require antibiotics and pesticides, and that doesn't come packaged in Styrofoam and plastic. You can select ingredients sourced from economies that uplift rather than impoverish their workers.

And the even better news is you can do so for totally selfish reasons. Because it turns out that the dietary pattern that aligns with all these altruistic goals is also the one that will give you the best odds for a long and healthy life.

Wouldn't it be horrible if we had to choose between our health and the health of other people and the environment? What a quandary that would put us in!

But thankfully, we can do our part to bring about a vision of healthy, ethical, and sustainable food for all while enjoying delicious meals and nourishing the best versions of ourselves. Enjoying real superfoods is definitely a win-win!

And as you're about to discover, it can also be utterly delicious.

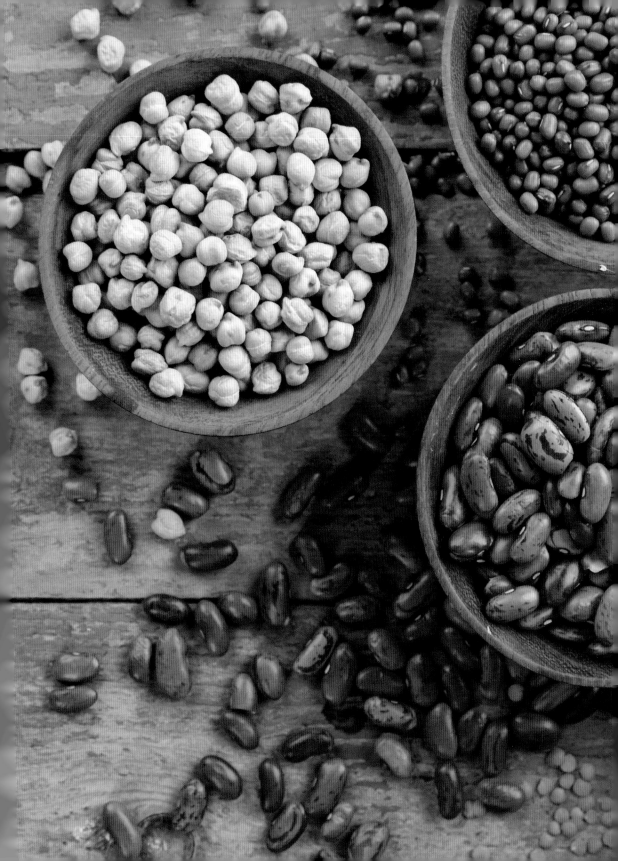

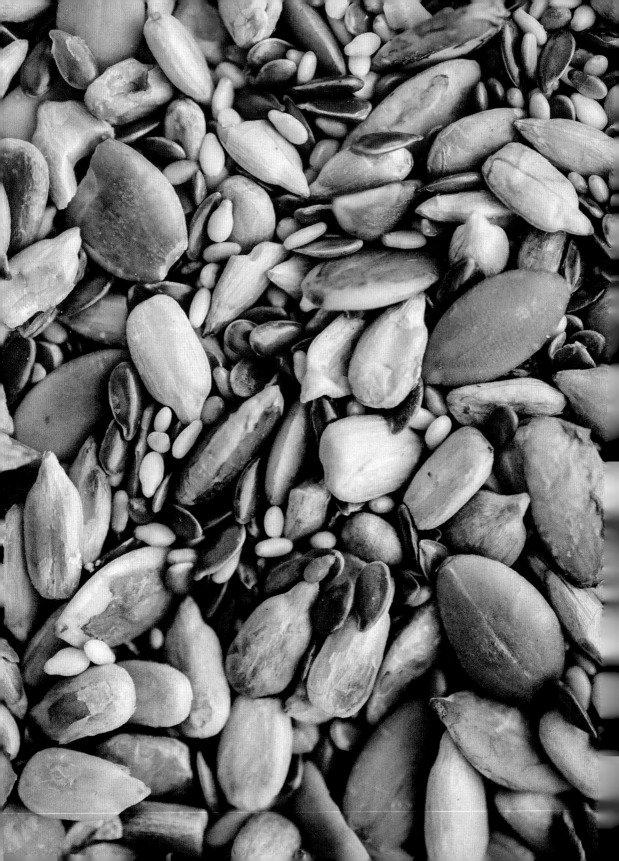

HOW TO USE THIS COOKBOOK

It's my hope that this cookbook will serve as a guide—a compendium of accessible, nutrient-packed foods you can keep in your meal rotations to optimize or improve your health.

The first section introduces the real superfoods and shares their nutritional powers, documented health benefits, types and varieties, and general guidance about how to incorporate them into your diet. Each chapter focuses on a different category of superfood and includes a mini-index to all the recipes that feature that category, so you can interrupt your reading to go make a meal or snack at your convenience.

The second section features recipes by Nichole Dandrea-Russert, MS, RDN, the culinary manager here at Food Revolution Network. Nichole presents over 60 mouthwatering recipes, each of which features multiple categories of the real superfoods. You get a wide range of dishes that cover breakfast, lunch, and dinner; salads, soups, and stews; sides, snacks, and desserts; and drinks.

You can read the book cover to cover or just sample individual chapters. If you like, you can even skip the entire first section (it's okay, even though I worked hard on it!) and jump immediately to the recipes. I hope you'll use this book often, and work it hard. (Some of my favorite cookbooks are so full of food stains, they're practically scratch and sniff at this point.)

I also hope you'll become an ambassador for real superfoods. That might mean posting images and videos of the dishes you make on Instagram or TikTok (or whatever social media platform is the next hot thing), or simply sharing healthy and delicious meals with friends and neighbors.

And remember that Nichole, as talented as she is, doesn't have a monopoly on recipe creation. **Let her creativity spark your own,** as you discover new and exciting ways to get these amazing real superfoods onto your plate and into your body.

Your body will thank you for the rest of your life. Enjoy!

OCEAN ROBBINS

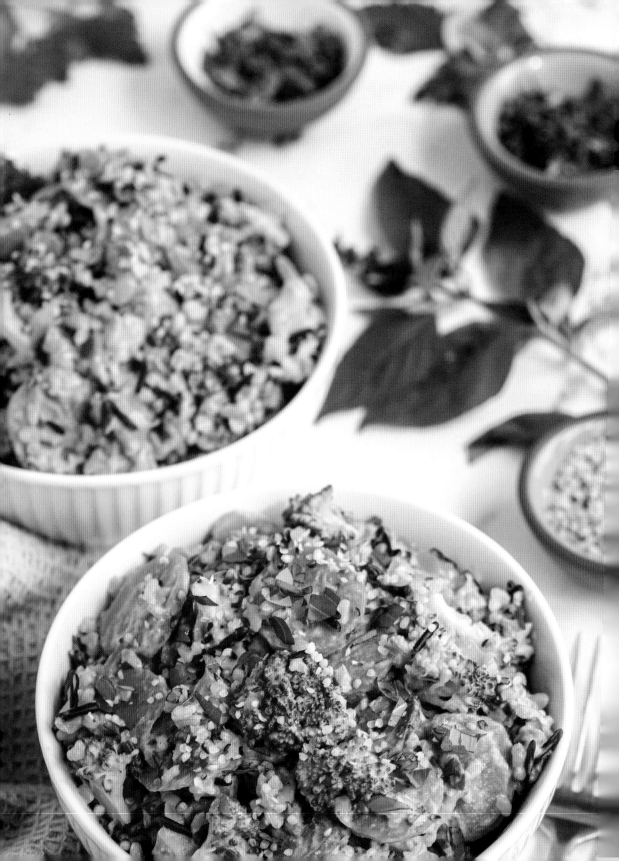

PART ONE

REAL SUPERFOODS

CHAPTER 1

LEAFY GREENS

When I was a kid, I ate kale at least 150 days a year. It was so important to us that my folks, proud hippies that they were, almost named me Kale.

Every fall, we'd get a huge delivery of all the staples that would carry us through the coming year. Fresh fruit and vegetables, nuts and seeds, whole and ground grains, legumes, dry goods, herbs and spices. I remember the days that followed as a brief period of dizzying abundance; it was the only time I could eat most fruits, since few were suited to our island's soil and climate.

That truck also brought us the seeds for everything we grew in our garden. And the one plant that reliably survived the Canadian Pacific winters was Siberian kale. Not only survive but thrive: some biochemical magic rendered the leaves more tender and sweet when they'd been covered in snow.

For months at a time, kale was the one fresh thing we could eat, along with the cooked grains and legumes that made up the bulk of our winter calories. This was in the 1970s—long before kale became the poster child for healthy living.

By March, we hadn't exactly grown weary of kale, but we did long for variety. So we'd track the weather obsessively, wanting to get the spring seeds in the ground and growing as soon as we were reasonably sure that a surprise frost wouldn't destroy the crop.

One of our favorite crops was cabbage. From the tiny seeds that we buried in the soil and watered, we received an abundant harvest that was equal parts wonder, nutrition, and beauty. Throughout the spring, summer, and fall, we harvested and feasted on a variety of greens: lettuces and cabbages,

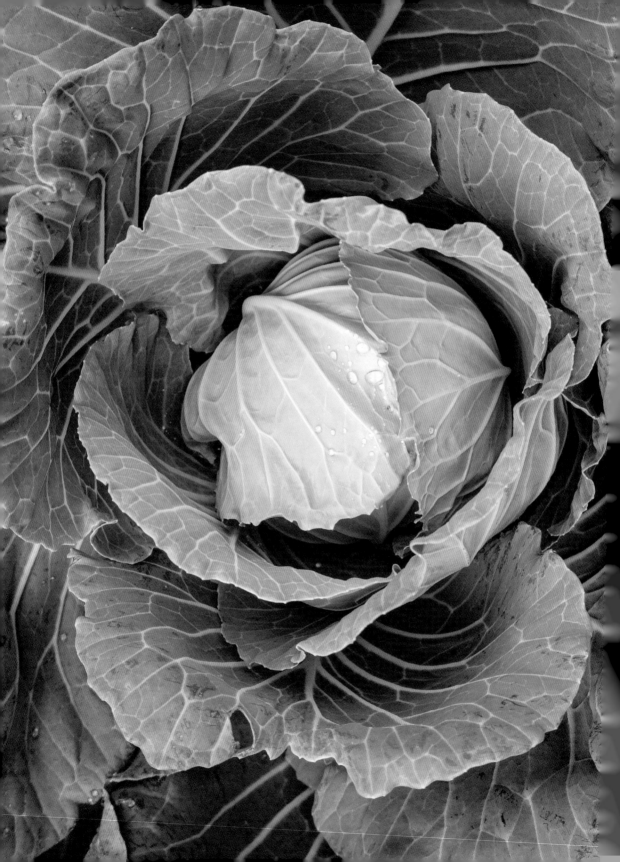

heads and leaves, mild and bitter (yes, I'm talking about you, mustard!).

We ate simply but well. Mostly we just steamed our greens, adding a drizzle of tamari and a few drops of olive oil, or some cayenne pepper and nutritional yeast if we were feeling fancy. And the vitality of those greens always lifted us.

While some plants can be finicky in a garden, greens are among the easiest plants to grow. It's as if they really want to do well and thrive. They'll put up with a lot, and even, like that Siberian kale, taste better in response to adversity.

The resiliency of greens reminds me of the resiliency of the human spirit, which also can rise in amazing ways in hard times. I learned recently that seeds for collard greens and okra were brought from their native Africa to the American South — woven into the braids of enslaved women and girls. Those courageous women sowed the seeds into the new yet not unfamiliar soils of Georgia, Mississippi, and South Carolina.

Many traditions honor greens as the literal and symbolic harbingers of springtime, of renewal, of a return to vibrant life after a long, hard winter. They're as varied as life itself: some are sweet and mild, and some have a kick to them. Some are tender and some are tough. And a diet that includes a variety of greens can help you remain vital and alive throughout the seasons of your life.

Why Leafy Greens?

One way to think about the ideal human diet is to look at what we have evolved to eat. The paleo story emphasizes "man as hunter," which is only part of the story (and a tad sexist at that). Archeologists studying past civilizations and anthropologists observing most modern-day hunter-gatherer peoples agree that the majority of calories and nutrients in the human diet come from plants, not animals.

It makes sense. Unlike animals, plants don't run away or fight back. You can eat from many plants without killing them, which is really convenient if you want to come back and do it again later.

And of all the parts of a plant, leaves would likely be the most accessible. While plants typically fruit only for a short season, they may have leaves much of the year. And unlike roots, leaves are right there in the open for all to see.

From our modern perspective, leaves (or "leafy greens," which is how we'll refer to them from now on) are an ideal food. They're rich in many of the nutrients we need in order to thrive. And they're low in calories, which is why horses have to spend up to 20 hours a day eating grass.

Actually, I have to qualify one statement I just made: that plants don't fight back. And I'm not just talking about poison ivy. While plants are delighted to have animals—including us—eat their fruits (which is why they make them colorful and sweet) and spread their seeds, they're not crazy about predators scarfing down all their leaves, which they need to make the food for their own seeds. And one way they protect their leaves from predators is to make each one a tiny bit toxic.

You might think that mild toxicity would be a bad thing, nutritionally speaking. But it turns out that in the case of most leafy greens, it's the opposite, thanks to a concept called hormesis. Basically, hormesis means that some kinds of stress, in low doses, are good for us. Just as the stress of having to lift a heavy weight will break down your muscle fibers so they grow back bigger and stronger, having to deal with small amounts of plant toxins may actually stimulate our immune systems and make us healthier. That's one theory, anyway, about why the antioxidants that plants produce both to repel leaf-eaters and to protect their tissues from sun damage are so good for us.

And in a bit, we'll see what science has discovered about the health benefits of leafy greens. Spoiler alert: they really do deserve to be the subject of the first chapter of a superfoods book. First, though, let's get clear on what leafy greens we're talking about.

Types of Leafy Greens

Leafy greens come in five distinct families: cruciferous, taproot, lettuce, chicory, and amaranth.

Some of the most widely available cruciferous greens include arugula, kale, bok choy, cabbage, collards, and mustard greens. This family is known for a mega-powerful cancer-fighting compound, sulforaphane.

You're probably more used to eating the taproots than their greens, but radish greens, beet greens, carrot tops, celeriac greens, and turnip greens are all nutritional powerhouses, and—prepared skillfully—pretty darn tasty. The nice thing about these greens is that you can think of them as bonuses if you're already growing or buying the roots.

The lettuce greens include all varieties of lettuce, the most common being iceberg and romaine. But more and more people are now enjoying other types, including red leaf, Butterhead, Bibb, Boston, and oak.

The chicory family of greens consists of lettuce's artsy and temperamental cousins, and they are both heartier and more bitter than most lettuce varieties. Part of the dandelion branch of the sunflower family, the most commonly consumed chicory greens include endive (which you can pronounce "enn-dive" or "on-deev," depending on whether you want to sound down-home or fancy), and frisée, which you pronounce "free-zay," and never "frisbee."

Amaranth family greens include well-known species like spinach and Swiss chard, as well as greens from the amaranth plant itself, which is better known for its tiny cereal grains and its brightly colored, catkin-like flower clusters.

Technically, there's a sixth family, the green herbs, but they'll have to wait until the Herbs and Spices chapter to get their due.

You may have noticed that most but not all the leafy greens mentioned above are in fact green. Let's talk about that for a minute. The reason most leaves are green has to do with an amazing chemical that plants make: chlorophyll. It has two main functions. First, it's an antioxidant that protects plants from oxidative stress. Second, it turns sunlight into energy, a technological feat that puts Star Trek's replicator to shame.

It turns out that chlorophyll doesn't turn all the sunlight into energy, though. It does a great job with blue spectrum light, which it absorbs greedily. But it can't do much with green spectrum light, which it rejects. It's kind of weird and cool when you think about it: leaves look green to us when in fact green is the only color they don't absorb (and therefore bounce back).

What about the non-green leaves? Well, some plants manufacture other health-boosting antioxidants, and these are most commonly red, purple, or orange. Depending on the ratio of these compounds to chlorophyll, a leaf could be reddish, such as certain varieties of Swiss chard or lettuce, or purple, as in the inaccurately named red cabbage. It's kind of cool that you can get a clue about their health benefits from their hue, don't you think?

Leafy Greens Nutrition

All leafy greens, even the much-maligned iceberg lettuce, are packed with carotenoids and antioxidants. Many contain dietary nitrates, which we'll see below are natural vasodilators and therefore good for the cardiovascular system (that's the heart, lungs, and circulatory system to you and me). Leafy greens are also rich in B vitamins; vitamins A, E, and K; and minerals like calcium, iron, and magnesium.

Leafy greens are really low in calories because they consist largely of two calorie-free components: fiber and water. Raw kale delivers under 200 calories per pound (and a pound is a heck of a lot of kale to eat in one sitting—believe me, I know). More water-rich greens like lettuces contain half that many calories per pound. And roughly one-third of those calories are in the form of protein.

LEAFY GREENS FAMILY	NUTRIENTS	SERVING SIZE
Cruciferous Cauliflower Kale Broccoli Arugula/Rocket Brussel Sprouts Cabbage Bok Choy Collards Mustard Greens	Vitamin A/Beta-carotene, Lutein • Zeaxanthin Antioxidants • Folate Niacin (B3) • Pantothenic acid (B5) • Pyridoxine (B6) Vitamin C • Vitamin K Vitamin E • Copper Magnesium • Potassium Fiber • Zinc	Cooked: 1–1½ cup (124 g–186 g) Raw: 2–2½ cups (40 g–54 g)
Taproots Carrots Beets Radishes Parsnips Turnips Kohlrabi Rutabaga	Beta-carotene Fiber • Folate Pyridoxine (B6) Vitamin C • Iron Manganese • Potassium Copper	Cooked: 1–1½ cup (145 g–217 g) Raw: ½–1 cup (64 g–128 g)
Lettuces Butter Cress Iceberg Mache Mesclun Romaine Spinach	Vitamin A/Beta-carotene, Lutein • Zeaxanthin Antioxandants • Folate Panthothenic acid (B5) Vitamin C • Vitamin K Copper • Magnesium Potassium	Cooked: 1–1½ cup (180 g–270 g) Raw: 2–2½ cups (60 g–80 g)
Chicory Endive Radicchio Escarole Frisée Dandelion Greens	Vitamin A/Beta-carotene, Lutein, Zeaxanthin Antioxandants • Folate Panthothenic acid (B5) Vitamin C • Vitamin K Copper • Magnesium Potassium • Fiber Zinc	Cooked: 1–1½ cup (105 g–158 g) Raw: 2–2½ cups (210 g–263 g)
Amaranth Joseph's Coat Chinese Spinach Callaloo Vleeta Chaulai (Indian Spinach)	Vitamin A • Vitamin C Vitamin K • Folate Pyridoxine (B6) Potassium • Calcium Iron • Manganese Zinc	Cooked: 1–1½ cup (132g–198g) Raw: 1½–2 cups (42 g–56 g)

The Evidence

Before we dive into what the studies tell us, there's one important thing you should know: very few people are eating leafy greens on a regular basis. And that means we don't have much evidence for the health benefits of, say, three or more servings a day. So pretty much all the data we have to work with is based on the differences between people literally avoiding all leafy greens (like, they remove the iceberg leaf from their sandwich) and people eating an average of 1.3 servings per day.

To help you see how a range that narrow can make it seem that leafy greens aren't as big a deal as they probably are, imagine that instead of nutrition, we're trying to figure out the effect of speed on injury and mortality in car crashes. And we study three groups of crash tests: those standing still, those driving into a brick wall at 5 miles per hour, and those going 10 miles per hour. In each case, there are zero injuries and no deaths from cars colliding at those speeds. So the researchers might conclude, "Speed has no effect on the risk of injury or death." Of course, had they looked at crash tests at speeds of 35, 50, or 75 miles per hour, they would have found a direct cause-and-effect relationship.

That's all to say, whatever we know about the health benefits of leafy greens consumption, they're probably much greater and more profound than we are currently measuring. That said, let's look at the evidence that leafy greens deserve their superfood designation.

The Super Health Benefits of Leafy Greens

Whether you just want to live a long, healthy life or you're hoping to make it until Silicon Valley figures out how to ensure your immortality by uploading your brain to the cloud, a diet rich in leafy greens can help—a lot.

Leafy Greens Fight Cancer

All leafy greens provide antioxidants that suppress the initiation, growth, and proliferation of cancer cells by resisting and repairing cell damage.[1] The best-studied greens in this regard are the cruciferous greens, thanks in large part to sulforaphane.[2] As you can see in the name, sulforaphane contains sulfur, which is the funky-smelling compound responsible for the smell of rotten eggs. And just as the sulfur compounds protect plants from pests, they also protect our cells from inflammation and oxidation.

The fiber in leafy greens also protects against cancers of the digestive system, and possibly some forms of breast cancer as well. This might be because fiber helps move food and waste through the body more quickly, reducing our exposure to toxins. Eating lots of fiber is also a good way to stay slim, and this is important because being overweight is a risk factor for at least 12 types of cancer.

Leafy Greens Protect Your Brain

If you want to avoid cognitive decline and dementia, a daily serving of leafy greens (or more!) could be your new best friend. A study from Rush University in Chicago looked at the relationship between diet and brain health in 1,000 people over the age of 58.[3] The researchers divided participants into 5 quintiles based on how many servings of leafy greens they consumed per day.

The lowest quintile ate, on average, 0.09 servings a day. Given that a serving was deemed to be ½ cup of cooked greens or 1 cup of raw greens, this means that they ate less than 2 grams per day. You know what weighs 2 grams? A US dime, a single cashew, or a plastic sandwich bag.

The highest quintile group, on the other hand, consumed an average of 1.3 servings a day, which isn't that much either (1.3 servings of raw kale is 27 grams, which is the same weight as a pencil or 6 sheets of paper).

Okay, so that was a fairly elaborate setup. And here's the stunning punchline: the group that ate a pencil's worth of leafy greens were functionally 11 years younger than the dime group. And this was based on a battery of cognitive tests conducted over an average of five years.

The heroic chemical in leafy greens most responsible for slowing cognitive decline appears to be lutein (and to a lesser extent, its sister-compound zeaxanthin).[4] We've known from autopsy studies that lutein is the dominant carotenoid antioxidant in the brain. The brain is a fatty organ, and one thing that happens to fat is that it goes rancid. Lutein and zeaxanthin combat fat rancidity that can be caused by oxidation and the brain's high metabolic turnover.

Once scientists discovered how to measure concentrations of lutein in the human brain without having to dissect it (which obviously defeats the purpose of resisting cognitive decline), they discovered that lutein levels correlated with cognitive performance across lifespan, from centenarians down to toddlers. Lutein also correlates with visual and auditory acuity (meaning, the ability to see and hear well).

While most leafy greens are good sources of lutein and zeaxanthin, the big winners here are kale (26,000 mcg per serving)[5] and spinach (36,000 mcg per serving).[6]

Leafy Greens Fight Type 2 Diabetes

Leafy greens protect against type 2 diabetes through a number of different mechanisms. The fiber in leafy greens stabilizes blood sugar by slowing down the absorption of dietary sugars into the bloodstream. Foods high in fiber and water also make you feel full, so you don't overeat. And overconsumption of calories is one of the biggest behavioral risk factors for development of type 2 diabetes. The vitamins in leafy greens, along with the mineral magnesium, also help regulate blood sugar.

One study showed that 1½ daily servings of leafy greens can cut your diabetes risk by 14 percent.[7]

Leafy Greens Protect Your Heart

Here's a case where the evidence may dramatically undersell the benefit. The majority of studies exploring the connection between leafy green consumption and cardiovascular health just look at spinach and lettuce, the two most common greens in the modern Western diet. Even with that limitation, most studies find that greens reduce the risk of cardiovascular disease.[8] For the greatest protection, researchers recommend eating 120 grams per day, which comes out to about 4 cups of raw spinach or just under 1 cup of cooked red cabbage.

Greens that deserve special mention in the heart-protecting department are those high in nitrates, including spinach, arugula, kale, and cabbage. Your body converts the nitrates into nitric oxide, which is a signaling molecule that tells your blood vessels to dilate. More and more endurance athletes are "doping" with nitric oxide–rich foods such as beets, beet greens, and beet juice to help their cardio systems work more efficiently. But even if you aren't planning to rock a triathlon or Spartan race any time soon, that vasodilation can lower your blood pressure, which prevents plaque buildup in your arteries and enables your heart to circulate blood with less effort.

How to Choose Leafy Greens

When buying leafy greens, look for fresh, firm leaves and bright colors. Avoid greens that look wilted or have yellow or brown spots. They should also pass the "sniff test" and either not smell at all or give off an aroma that's similar to the plant's characteristic taste. For example, arugula's sharp scent is redolent of pepper. If it smells like moldy socks, that's probably not a good sign.

Store greens in the refrigerator, unwashed, and rinse and dry them just before using. You can keep them wrapped in produce bags, with all the air burped out, or store them in an airtight container. Most do well in the fridge's crisper drawer. Hardy leaves like kale and collards will last longer than lettuces or bok choy, but why wait? Try to eat leafy greens within a couple of days, so you never have to look down on a sad, slimy plastic bag full of organic matter decomposing behind the oat milk and tub of hummus.

Cabbage, on the other hand, lasts a really long time in the fridge. You may be able to store a head in the crisper drawer for up to several weeks. Store any unused chunks in an airtight container to prevent decay.

How to Prepare Leafy Greens

You can serve leafy greens raw, cooked, or fermented. Each way has its own nutritional benefits and taste profiles, so you may need to experiment to find your favorite ways to prepare them.

Raw Greens

The most popular raw greens include lettuces, cabbages (shredded, in slaw), and sharp salad greens like arugula and mizuna. Serve them in salads, add them to sandwiches, or use them as toppings on main dishes and grains. You can tenderize stemmed and chopped collards and kale by massaging the leaves with avocado before tossing them with other salad ingredients. Arugula also makes a delicious, peppery pesto. Because collard greens hold together well, they make an excellent wrap material if you want to avoid processed wraps made with flour.

Green Smoothies

One easy way to consume lots of raw greens like kale, spinach, and arugula—and even herbs like parsley, cilantro, and lovage—is to blend them into green smoothies. You can use fresh or frozen greens for smoothies. The trick to great smoothies is to add just enough fruit to make it sweet (and if you're feeding kids or picky eaters, to mask the taste of the greens).

Chips

Kale chips might be considered raw by purists, depending on how you dehydrate them. Wash, de-rib, and massage the kale with some seasonings, and dry away! You can use a dedicated dehydrator or just warm them on baking trays in the oven for a couple of hours.

Dips

Raw greens like spinach and kale make great dip ingredients. You can add them to a food processor or blender when making hummus and nondairy cheese spreads.

Boiling or Steaming

If you aren't going to use the water you cooked them in, steaming your greens is better than boiling them because more nutrients remain in the greens instead of leaching out into the water. Steamed greens may seem bland, but they can be a wonderful part of a macrobiotic-inspired plate—served with a grain and some legumes, tofu, or tempeh, and covered in a piquant ginger sauce. The best time to boil greens is if you're going to make them into soup, which enables you to drink the nutrients that end up in the water.

Baking, Roasting, or Grilling

Head cabbages hold together well even after you slice them, and you can cut them into pieces of equal size to be baked, roasted, or grilled. The longer they cook, the sweeter and more tender they become.

Stir-Frying

Stir-frying can be a tasty way to prepare greens that even picky eaters will enjoy—and it can be healthy, too, as long as you don't smother your veggies in overheated oil. The healthiest way to stir-fry greens (and other veggies, for that matter) may be to omit the oil entirely. To stir-fry oil free, you can use water, broth, soy sauce, or liquid soy or coconut aminos to keep the veggies from sticking to the pan and burning. Stir constantly (as Martin Yan, the chef on *Yan Can Cook* reminds us, "It's stir-fry, not stare-fry!"), and don't overheat the pan. A pro trick is to stir-fry some onions first in a dry pan and add liquid just when they start to caramelize and brown. The sugars from the onion will make for a rich, flavorful sauce even before you add a "real" sauce to the leafy greens dish.

Fermented Greens

Another great way to enjoy greens is to ferment them. You can make sauerkraut and kimchi from head cabbages, as well as leafy brassicas like bok choy and napa cabbage. Fermenting is a good way to add all-important probiotics to your diet, which will make your gut microbes very happy.

LEAFY GREENS RECIPES

BREAKFAST

Elixir of Life Smoothie Bowl

Rockin' Rollup Lentil Sausage Breakfast Wraps

Easy Peasy Tofu Breakfast Bites

No Muss, No Fuss Breakfast Burrito

MAINS

Simple Tri-Color Umami Stir-Fry

Pile 'Em High Black Bean Tostadas

Sprout and Flourish Grain Bowl

(Bring La) Fiesta Roasted Sweet Potato Bowl

Everyday Lentil Lunch

Kickin' Kimchi "Fried" Rice and Veggies

Everything but the Kitchen Sink Potato Nachos

SALADS

Fill Me with Warmth Tempeh and Kale Salad

Uncomplicated Crunchy Kale Slaw

Feeling Upbeet and Lively Lentil Salad

Super Seed Autumn Salad with Tart Pomegranate Dressing

SOUPS/STEWS

Perfectly Spiced Spinach Lentil Soup

Butter Bean Me Up One-Pot Soup

Sweet and Savory Peanut Soup

Simple-to-Make Supergreen Mushroom and Potato Soup

Creamy Dreamy Arugula and White Bean Soup

SIDES

Slow-Cooked Rainbow Collards

Herbaceous Wild Rice and Mushroom Stuffing

SNACKS

Zesty Chili Lime Kale Chips

DRINKS

Invigorating Tropical Green Smoothie

Purple Paradise Smoothie

CHAPTER 2

MUSHROOMS

There were mushrooms growing in the old-growth cedar forest on the island where I grew up. Some were certainly edible, but I was warned of the dangers of wild harvesting if you weren't an expert mycologist, so I didn't bring any home to eat. What I harvested, instead, was the earthy aroma of the fungi and the felt sense that the earth beneath my feet was teeming with life.

And I've learned since that fungi are a kind of energetic bridge between plant and animal life. They are the great recyclers of the planet, breaking down the dead and dying so that the building blocks of biochemistry can be shared with new life.

For a long time, the only member of the fungus kingdom stocked by standard Western grocery stores was white button mushrooms. You could get them whole or sliced, fresh or canned. Nobody thought of them as a superfood; they were white, a color that we interpret as signifying a lack of nutritional merit.

Then the Western wellness world discovered a treasure trove of edible fungi that many households, particularly Asian ones, had been using for many years: richly hued mushrooms such as shiitake and maitake, along with other colorful and edible fungi like Cordyceps, lion's mane, and Chaga. Researchers called these mushrooms "functional foods," with positive benefits to our health beyond their vitamins and minerals. Some have been used for centuries in traditional Chinese medicine, Indian Ayurveda, and other cultural traditions to help defend the body against physical, chemical, and biological stressors.

When scientists discovered that certain compounds known as aromatase inhibitors, found in many edible mushrooms,

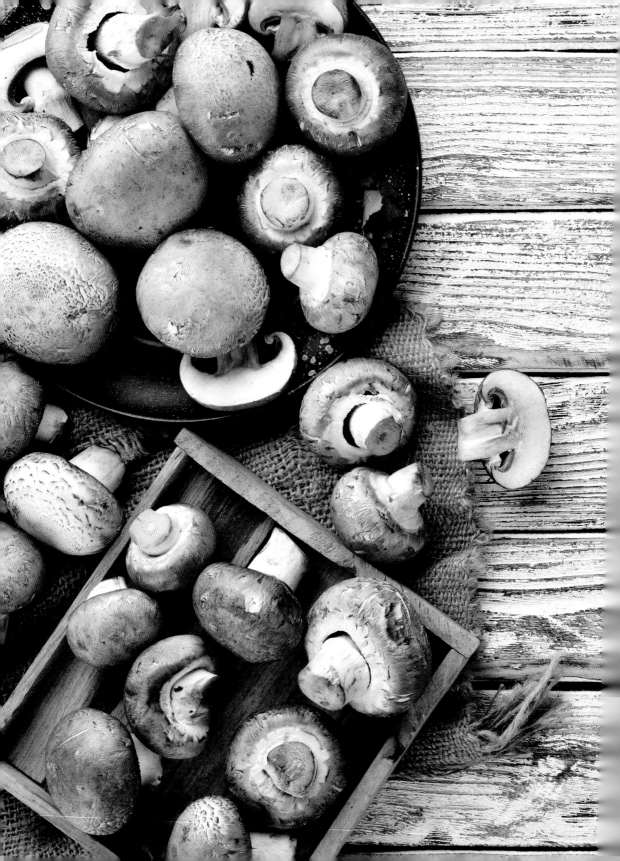

could help inhibit the development of breast cancer, they immediately became curious. Which mushroom would prove most powerful? Wood ear? Oyster? Shiitake? Chanterelle?

In 2001, an immunology lab in California announced the winner: regular old white button mushrooms.[1]And the bigger the mushroom, the stronger the effect. That's right—white button mushrooms are an amazing superfood. And so are many other edible, medicinal, and adaptogenic mushrooms that are becoming ever more popular and readily available in mainstream commerce and culture.

What Are Mushrooms?

First, let's clear up any confusion about definitions. Mushrooms are members of the fungi kingdom and are not the same as plants. In fact, fungi are more closely related to animals than plants; like us, they don't photosynthesize. The compound that provides structure to fungi's cell walls is chitin, which makes up the exoskeletons of lobsters and ants and the scales of fish.

Mushrooms are the fruiting bodies of fungi in the same way that a pear is the fruiting body of a pear tree. They're made up of three parts: the stipe (stem), the pileus (cap), and the lamellae (gills). The "seeds" of the mushroom "fruit" are its spores, which form a network of microscopic rooting threads called mycelium. This is a mass of threadlike branches that mushrooms use

to decompose nearby plant material in order to extract nutrients. A mycelium can live for many years, communicating with plants and sending up its annual crop of mushrooms.

The mycelium can be small and compact or can span underground over thousands of acres with mushrooms popping up out of the ground sporadically or in clusters. The world's largest organism is thought to be a mycelium network belonging to a mushroom technically called *Armillaria ostoyae*, commonly known as the honey mushroom, found in Malheur National Forest, Oregon. How enormous is it? This mushroom's mycelium network covers two square miles and is around 8,650 years old. So if you ever get tired of knock-knock jokes, you can try this riddle: "What's two and a half miles across, 8,650 years old, and lives in Oregon?"

Types of Mushrooms

In addition to white button mushrooms, which are readily available and typically less expensive than other varieties (partly because it's possible to cultivate them commercially on a giant scale), there are many other kinds. Button, brown cremini, and portobello mushrooms are the same variety, just aged longer or allowed to grow bigger (buttons are the youngsters, brown cremini are the teens, and portobello are the grown-ups).

Mushroom Nutrition

You'll find different kinds and ratios of nutrients in different mushroom varieties, so for this section, I'll focus exclusively on that surprising superfood, white button mushrooms (since they're generally the most affordable of the fungi). They're low calorie and a source of protein. They're loaded with antioxidants—beating out such formidable plant foods as tomatoes, green peppers, pumpkins, zucchini, carrots, and green beans—and even topping more expensive shiitake and oyster mushrooms.

Button mushrooms are also packed with vitamins and minerals like B vitamins, selenium, potassium, and copper. They contain two types of important dietary fibers, beta-glucans and chitin. Interestingly, when mushrooms are exposed to sunlight while growing, they are one of the few natural dietary sources of vitamin D.

Why White Button Mushrooms Deserve Superfood Status

Okay, this is where I have to remind myself that this is just a chapter, not an entire book. Science has discovered over 200 conditions affecting human health that can be treated to some extent with mushrooms, and at least 100 mechanisms by which mushrooms support our health. So what follows is in no way all encompassing.

Mushrooms Can Improve Your Gut Health

Mushrooms are a gut-friendly food,[2] offering the good bacteria in your gut lots of prebiotic[3] fiber. They've also been found[4] to balance the microbiome's beneficial bacteria, such as acidophilus and bifidobacterium.

Mushrooms Can Protect Your Heart

One of the amino acids found in mushrooms, ergothioneine, has been associated with a lower risk of heart disease. In a study concluded in 2019 (started in 1998), researchers measured 112 different aspects of blood chemistry of over 3,000 people who didn't have heart disease at the start of the study, and then followed them for an average of 21 years. The blood marker that best predicted continued freedom from heart disease was ergothioneine. The researchers concluded that a diet high in ergothioneine-rich foods was a good way to obtain that protection.[5]

Mushrooms Can Support Your Brain Health

Several studies have shown that eating mushrooms can help protect your brain. In 2017, Japanese researchers analyzed a 2006 population study and discovered a linear relationship between mushroom consumption and lower incidences of dementia.[6] And this relationship held even when eliminating other factors that might also support brain health, like consumption of fruits and vegetables and educational level attained.

In 2019, a research team in Singapore found that eating two servings of mushrooms lowered the risk of mild cognitive decline (MCI) by 43 percent. That's huge since brain researchers see MCI as an intermediate step on the way to dementia.[7]

Mushrooms Can Help Prevent Cancer

Roughly one in nine women will develop breast cancer during her lifetime. While early detection and medical advances have improved survival rates, it's still a terrifying diagnosis for many people. And early detection is not the same as prevention. What if there were a food that could help reduce the risk?

Can you picture a regular white button mushroom? Now imagine cutting that single mushroom in half, and then cooking and eating it. And having just that much mushroom, every day.

Congratulations! In that modest thought experiment, you just cut your risk of developing breast cancer by two thirds. You read that right—a study of over 2,000 Chinese women found that eating just a third of an ounce of (about a half of one) mushroom daily cut the risk of breast cancer by 64 percent.[8]

Men shouldn't feel left out; white button mushrooms have been shown to lower blood levels of prostate-specific antigen (PSA), a marker associated with the development of prostate cancer.[9] They may do this by suppressing androgen receptors, thereby slowing the growth of cancer cells.

Mushrooms Can Support Your Immune System

Mushrooms enhance the ability of dendritic cells, found in bone marrow, to produce T cells that kill disease-causing pathogens.[10] They are also a rich source of compounds called beta-glucans, which activate white blood cells to help fight off foreign substances and diseases.

Mushrooms Can Support Your Digestive and Metabolic Health

The more fiber you eat, the lower your chances of developing type 2 diabetes, according to a giant meta-analysis published in *The Lancet* in early 2019.[11] And mushrooms are one of the best sources of fiber out there. In particular, they contain lots of prebiotic fiber, which is yummy food for the "good" gut bacteria that do incredibly important jobs in your body. And a healthy gut is one of the best defenses against literally dozens of maladies, including type 2 diabetes and digestive disorders such as irritable bowel syndrome.

MUSHROOM TYPE	BENEFITS
White (button, portobello, and cremini)	Supports healthy immune function Rich in antioxidants • Antiaging • Anticancer Supports healthy brain function and cognition Heart healthy • Supports healthy digestion
Shiitake	Supports healthy immune function • Heart healthy • Lowers cholesterol • Maintains healthy blood pressure • Rich in antioxidants
Enoki	Supports healthy immune function • Anticancer • Heart healthy • Support healthy brain function and cognition • Rich in antioxidants
Lion's Mane	Supports healthy immune function • Focus, mental clarity, and mood • Reduces anxiety symptoms • Anti-inflammatory Rich in antioxidants
Turkey Tail	Supports healthy immune function Anticancer • Rich in antioxidants
Hen of the Woods (maitake)	Supports healthy immune function Anticancer • Lowers cholesterol Blood sugar control • Anti-inflammatory
Beech (shimeji)	Supports healthy immune function • Rich in antioxidants Anti-inflammatory • Antimicrobial Lowers cholesterol • Heart healthy
Chanterelle	Supports healthy immune function Rich in antioxidants • Supports bone health
Porcini	Supports healthy immune function Anti-inflammatory • Antiviral/antibacterial Supports healthy digestion • Reduces risk of cardiovascular disease • Rich in antioxidants
Morel	Supports healthy immune function • Antitumor Anti-inflammatory • Rich in antioxidants
Oyster	Supports healthy immune function Reduces high blood pressure Lowers cholesterol • Blood sugar control • Healthy heart • Rich in antioxidants
Chaga	Supports healthy immune function • Reduces oxidative stress Rich in antioxidants • Anti-inflammatory • Lowers cholesterol Anticancer • Blood sugar control • Antitumor • Heart healthy

Mushrooms Can Help You with Weight Management

Eating more fiber is one of the most reliable ways to lose excess weight and keep it off. The modern industrialized diet is largely made up of animal products that contain no fiber and processed plant foods that have had the fiber removed. One of fiber's important functions is to make us feel full, so we stop eating before downing more calories than we need.

In one study, researchers asked some people to substitute mushrooms for meat in some of their recipes. Those who consumed at least 2.25 ounces of mushrooms per day (that's roughly 4 medium button mushrooms) experienced significantly more weight loss than those who didn't. They also ended up with a lower body mass index and a smaller waist circumference after one year.[12]

Culinary Uses for Edible Mushrooms

Mushrooms are a great substitute for meat in lots of dishes, thanks both to their strong umami flavor and meaty texture.

First, a word of caution: some edible mushrooms may contain a slightly toxic compound called agaritine. The good news is, agaritine breaks down when exposed to heat. So mushrooms should be cooked, not eaten raw.

Cooked mushrooms are delicious, and they're very easy to prepare in all sorts of ways. They're wonderful in stir-fries and casseroles. You can marinate and grill them, or slice them for a pizza topping. Mushroom soup is a classic; with an immersion blender, you can make it thick and comforting—a steaming anchor for a simple winter meal.

You can also use mushrooms as a basis for vegetarian burgers and other meat analogues.

However you choose to include mushrooms in your diet on a regular basis, your taste buds, your tummy, and your body as a whole will thank you!

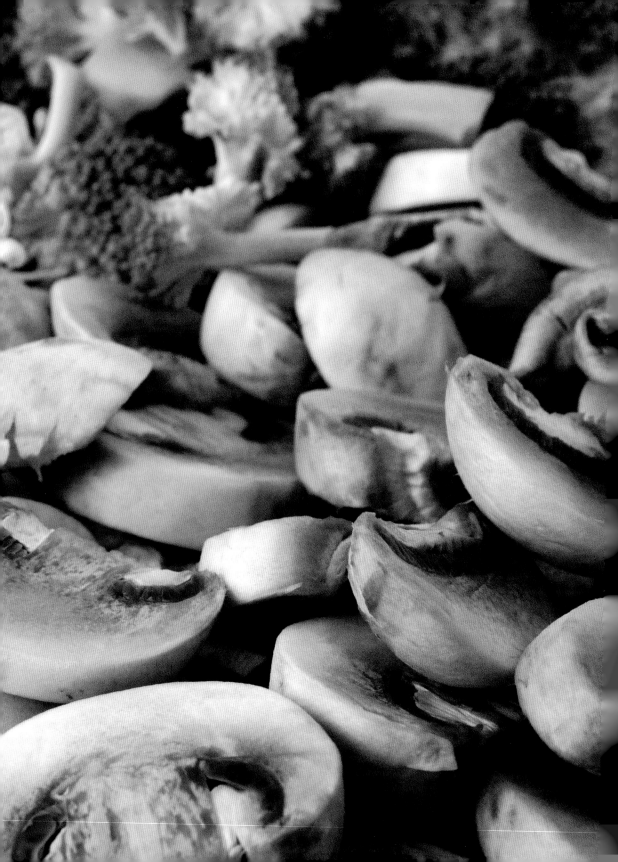

MUSHROOM RECIPES

BREAKFAST

Easy Peasy Tofu Breakfast Bites

MAINS

Simple Tri-Color Umami Stir-Fry

Plant-tastic Mushroom Ziti Bake

Built to Grill Beany Mushroom Burgers

Aromatic Veggie-Stuffed Acorn Squash

Nice 'n' Cheesy Comforting Casserole

Everyday Lentil Lunch

SALADS

Hearty Wild Rice, Mushroom, and Baby Broccoli Salad

SOUPS/STEWS

Simple-to-Make Supergreen Mushroom and Potato Soup

SIDES

Herbaceous Wild Rice and Mushroom Stuffing

CHAPTER 3

LEGUMES

When I was growing up, my folks and I probably got close to half our calories from legumes. Dried beans, peas, and lentils were the least expensive sources of macronutrients that we could get our hands on. When the September supply truck came, we would hoist the 25-pound bags of adzuki beans, pinto beans, black-eyed peas, and brown lentils into the cabin, feeling wealthy in the presence of such abundance.

And, boy, did we make good use of those legumes! We ate them in casseroles, in soups, in stews, in salads. We consumed legumes in mains and sides. We started sprouting legumes in mason jars decades before we found out that the practice enhanced the bioavailability of certain desirable nutrients and reduced concentrations of so-called "antinutrients" such as lectins. We just intuitively understood that making our food come alive was a good thing.

About eating legumes at practically every meal—that's actually a line from a rude verse I learned as a kid: "Beans, beans, they're good for your heart; the more you eat, the more you fart. The more you fart, the better you feel, so eat your beans with every meal."

I now have that earworm stuck in my head, which seems like it could get in the way of writing an inspiring chapter on legumes, a category of foods you might call "Beans and Friends." The only thing I can do is rewrite it in a more dignified manner:

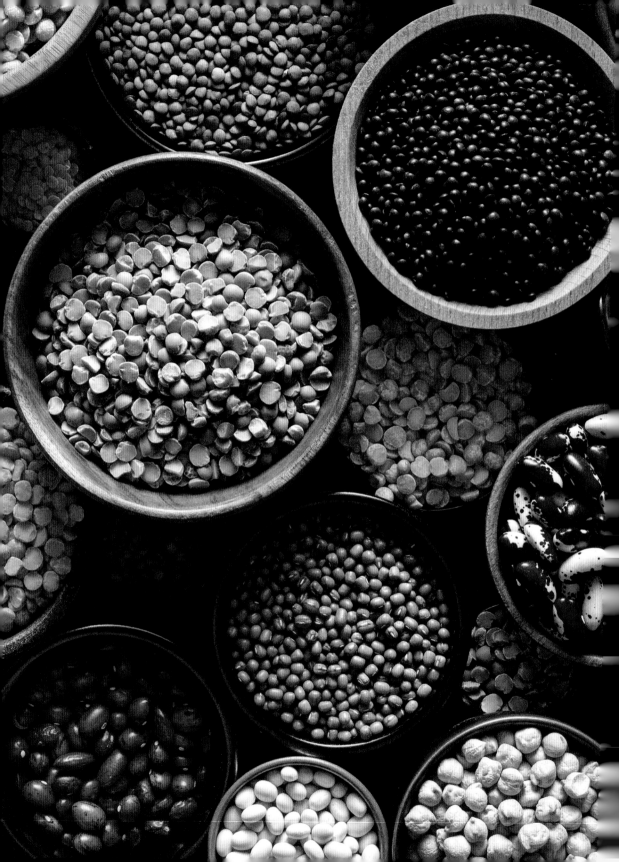

Beans, beans, they're good
for your heart,
Your brain, and your colon,
and that's just a start.
They help you lose weight;
they protect against cancer;
If long life is the question,
then beans are the answer.

Confession: I'm not sharing that poem just to impress you with my depth and sensitivity. I actually want to get that whole flatulence thing out of the way up front. In the rest of this chapter, you'll see that legumes are indeed a remarkable superfood; even that can of kidney beans in the back of your pantry is an incredibly nutritious powerhouse.

In fact, beans and other legumes are the food most tightly associated with a long life (in multiple studies across multiple populations around the world), and they're inexpensive, and they're delicious, and they're versatile—and most people aren't getting nearly enough. And the number one reason for that is: fear of breaking wind.

It's true that legumes can produce gas, especially if you're not used to them. Later, I'll tell you how to prepare them to minimize the "toot effect." But it turns out that their reputation as a wind machine is unfounded: A 2011 study surveyed people tasked with consuming ½ cup of legumes per day for 8 weeks. It found that between 80 and 90 percent experienced zero to one incident of increased flatulence or bloating

during that time. So if you, like me, can't put that old rhyme out of your mind, at least take it with a grain of salt as we explore the lustrous landscape of legumes.

What Are Legumes?

Gardeners love legumes because they do a neat trick: in partnership with bacteria in the soil, legumes take inert nitrogen from the air and make it accessible to the soil they grow in. That's one of the reasons George Washington Carver is honored for his contributions to the legume legacy; in addition to popularizing the peanut, he figured out that rotating soybeans into the planting cycle actually increased subsequent cotton yield.

There are four main types of legumes that we consume: beans, lentils, peas, and peanuts. Beans are generally the biggest of the three, often round, oval, or kidney-shaped. Common varieties include kidney, black, red, garbanzo (also known as chickpeas), cannellini, and lima beans. The most cultivated bean worldwide is the soybean, which you can consume fresh as edamame; in lightly processed foods such as tofu, tempeh, miso, and soymilk; and in more highly processed foods such as texturized vegetable protein and soybean oil.

BEANS/LEGUMES	SERVING	PROTEIN PER SERVING
Adzuki Beans	1 cup	17 grams
Black Beans	1 cup	14 grams
Black-Eyed Peas	1 cup	13 grams
Butter Beans	1 cup	12 grams
Cannellini Beans	1 cup	12 grams
Edamame (young soybeans)	1 cup	18 grams
Garbanzo Beans/Chickpeas	1 cup	11 grams
Green Peas	1 cup	8 grams
Great Northern Beans	1 cup	17 grams
Lentils	1 cup	18 grams
Pinto Beans	1 cup	12 grams
Red Beans/Small Kidney Beans	1 cup	14 grams
Split Peas	1 cup	16 grams
Tofu (extra firm)	4 ounces	16 grams

Lentils are smaller and lens-shaped (which is where they got their Latin name, *Lens culinaris* or "cooking lens"). Common lentils include brown, green, red, and yellow varieties.

Some peas, when split, look like lentils, but peas are their own kind of crop. They are round and grow in pods. Common varieties include green, yellow, and black-eyed peas.

And peanuts are their own category, which we're not going to cover here—because while they are technically legumes, I think of them as having the soul of a nut. (Possibly that's the origin of the name: "Hey, this pea tastes a lot like a nut. What shall we call it?")

Why Legumes Deserve Superfood Status

Beans, lentils, and peas differ somewhat in their nutritional profiles, but all edible legumes share some common features that make them highly valued dietary staples, especially among plant-based eaters.

Legumes are high in protein. In fact, for billions of people, legumes are their main source of the macronutrient, providing roughly one third of the world's total intake of protein. For example, a cup of cooked soybeans delivers 28 grams of protein, while a cup of lentils delivers 18, a cup of cooked garbanzos provides 16, and the same amount of black beans gives you 12 grams. (For perspective, the average 150-pound adult is generally thought to need 50 to 70 grams of protein per day.)

Legumes are high in fiber, especially resistant starch, which is the preferred food for many of the beneficial bacteria in your gut that do so much to keep you healthy. Garbanzo beans, for example, contain a whopping 13 grams of fiber per cup, which is more than many Americans get in an entire day, and which goes a long way toward filling your daily recommended intake of 40 grams or more.

Legumes are also an excellent source of essential minerals like iron, calcium, zinc, folate, potassium, magnesium, and choline, and they provide dozens of antioxidants, phytochemicals, and flavonoids that our bodies need to function optimally.

Legumes and Longevity

In 2000, Belgian demographer Michel Poulain was asked to contribute his expertise to an unusual study.[1] It appeared that the Italian island of Sardinia was home to a curiously large percentage of healthy centenarians, and researchers wanted to know why. Poulain was tasked with figuring out if the rumors were true; without strict record-keeping, it was a challenge to determine the year of someone's birth, especially if that year started with "18—."

Poulain threw himself into the work and soon discovered a particular part of the island where people, on average, lived the longest. He drew a blue line around this area and dubbed it the "Blue Zone."

Now that they had validated the data, the researchers began to search for explanations. One of the early hypotheses posited that high rates of intermarriage among a limited population coupled with very little immigration had selected for genetic resistance to diseases of aging. But with only one study population, it was going to be hard to generalize.

National Geographic reporter Dan Buettner heard about this research and figured it would make a great magazine story. Together with Poulain, he identified four other regions of the world—Okinawa, Japan; Nicoya, Costa Rica; Ikaria, Greece; and Loma Linda, California—that also produced remarkably long-lived and vibrant humans. Buettner's writing drew worldwide attention to the phenomenon, and soon the field of centenarian studies was rife with researchers seeking the secrets of these disparate "fountains of youth."

Eventually, they identified nine characteristics of all long-lived populations, including dietary and other lifestyle patterns. And the number one longevity food[2] in the world turned out to be . . . legumes. How about that—one of the world's least expensive foods also turns out to be the healthiest. Let's look at a few of the superfood properties of beans, peas, and lentils.

Legumes Fight Cancer

A study of over 2,000 adults[3] found that people who ate the most beans had a significantly reduced risk of a recurrence of colorectal polyps, which are precursors to colorectal cancer. Another study found that eating just two servings of legumes per week cut the risk of colon cancer in half.[4]

Garbanzo beans may deserve special mention here. Thanks to a rich concentration of particular compounds, garbanzos stimulate the production of a very important short-chain fatty acid called butyrate, which can reduce the risk of several cancers, including prostate, stomach, and colorectal.[5] And the fiber in beans can keep the digestive system moving at a healthy clip, which enables it to remove toxins before they can trigger breast cancer initiation or progression.[6]

Legumes Protect Your Brain

Legumes contain compounds that our brains use to make neurotransmitters, so it makes sense that eating them can preserve and even improve the health of the brain. A 2017 study[7] out of Italy showed that elderly people who started eating a lot of legumes not only didn't experience cognitive decline but actually improved their scores on a couple of cognitive tests.

And researchers from Rush University in Chicago found[8] that a dietary pattern heavy on legumes cut the risk of Alzheimer's in half compared to those who ate a standard modern diet heavy on animal products and processed foods.

Legumes Support Healthy Weight Management

If you're looking to maintain a healthy weight, legumes can help you there as well. A study in the *Journal of the American College of Nutrition* found that people who ate beans regularly had a 22 percent lower risk of obesity and were more likely to have a smaller waist than people who didn't eat beans.

It might be that, because beans are high in soluble fiber, they signal to your body that you're full and therefore should stop eating before you consume too many calories.[9]

Legumes Protect Your Heart

In a 2007 study,[10] researchers gave participants just ½ cup of pinto beans per day. After eight weeks, their total cholesterol dropped an average of nearly 20 points, and their LDL cholesterol levels dropped 14 points. There isn't a cholesterol-lowering drug on the market that can do better. More recent studies have shown that adding legumes to the diet, or, even better, replacing red meat with legumes, lowered total and LDL ("bad") cholesterol and triglyceride levels.

Legumes can also improve blood flow. Several studies found that a modest amount of legumes—less than a cup a day of cooked lentils or beans—lowered blood pressure significantly in just a few days.

Legumes Aid Your Digestion

All tooting jokes aside, beans and other legumes are great for moving things along and keeping you regular. Full of both prebiotic and probiotic fibers, they provide bulk to your stools so they can "float" easily through your large intestines and exit your body without straining.

Legumes Regulate Blood Sugar

All that fiber also keeps your blood sugar from spiking. One large population study found that people who ate garbanzo beans and hummus made from the beans had a much lower risk of developing metabolic syndrome, a suite of conditions linked both to cardiovascular disease and type 2 diabetes. Legumes have been shown to reduce both A1c and fasting blood glucose levels.[11] And for people with type 2 diabetes, a legume-rich diet helps manage the disease by stabilizing blood sugar.

How to Prepare and Serve Legumes

I don't know who needs to hear this, but you should definitely cook your dried legumes before eating them. Cooking breaks down so-called "antinutrients" (compounds that inhibit the absorption of other nutrients) like lectins and phytates. And cooking also eliminates toxins found in kidney beans. Plus, uncooked dried legumes can crack your teeth and are a real pain to chew—so just cook them!

To save time and energy, and to reduce the gassiness that beans can occasionally provoke in some people, you can soak your legumes before cooking. Cover the dried beans in room-temperature water for 12 to 48 hours, changing the water and rinsing 2 to 3 times a day. Give them a final rinse before putting them in fresh water and cooking thoroughly, until they're nice and tender.

My favorite way to cook legumes is in a pressure cooker. Not only does this method save even more time and energy, but the high pressure also allows water to penetrate the tough exterior of beans more fully, which makes them easily digestible.

Another way to render dried legumes edible is by sprouting them like we did when I was a kid. Soak them in water for 12 hours, then keep them moist using an upside-down mason jar with a screen lid or a dedicated sprouter, rinsing at least twice a day. After 2 to 4 days, the legume sprouts will be ready to eat cook and then eat—on sandwiches, in salads, or mixed into dips. Or you can also cook the sprouts if you prefer.

Culinary Uses for Legumes

Legumes add flavor, depth, and texture to many dishes. You can add cooked beans, peas, and lentils to salads, pasta dishes, grain bowls, stir-fries, soups, and stews. You can mash them into vegetarian burgers and meatballs, blend them into dips, and even use them in desserts to add bulk and nutrition. Black bean brownies might sound weird, but they can taste surprisingly amazing.

We can't talk about beans without mentioning hummus. This Middle Eastern spread that's found favor all over the world is traditionally made from garbanzo beans, but you can supplement with other beans or even swap out the garbanzos entirely (white beans work well; big butter beans can produce amazing creaminess). Hummus is incredibly versatile; it's a sandwich spread, a wrap filling, a salad dressing, a dip, and its very own side dish. I've even known a few people who will just sit down and eat it with a spoon (not that I'd know anything about that!).

The basic hummus template consists of just a few items: beans, a fat, an acid, and flavorings. Traditional hummus uses garbanzos, sesame tahini, lemon juice, salt, pepper,

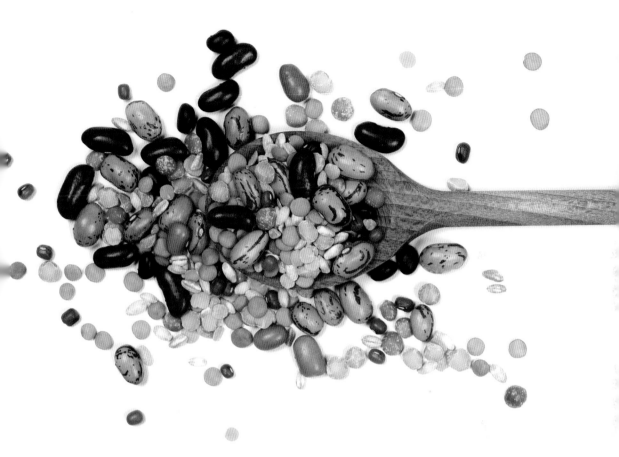

cumin, coriander, and garlic. Sometimes olive oil is included, as well. In addition to innovating with your choice of bean, you can use a nut butter instead of tahini, add vinegar in place of lemon juice, and spice it up however you like (Italian, Mexican, Thai—spin a globe and get inspired).

Soy is another culinary powerhouse. In addition to fresh, immature soybeans, called edamame in Japanese and increasingly available in Western supermarkets' frozen sections, you can also enjoy sprouted and pressure-cooked soybeans, or lightly processed soy products like tempeh and tofu, which take on whatever flavor they're cooked in. Tempeh, for example, makes a darn good bacon analogue when marinated in the right mix of spices and liquids. And tofu can substitute for scrambled eggs, ricotta, feta, and other cheeses, and lend creaminess and heft to soups, stews, and sauces.

LEGUMES RECIPES

BREAKFAST

Rockin' Rollup Lentil Sausage Breakfast Wraps
Easy Peasy Tofu Breakfast Bites
No Muss, No Fuss Breakfast Burrito
Comforting Cauliflower Lentil Kitchari

MAINS

Simple Tri-Color Umami Stir-Fry
Built to Grill Beany Mushroom Burgers
Aromatic Veggie-Stuffed Acorn Squash
Pile 'Em High Black Bean Tostadas
Nice 'n' Cheesy Comforting Casserole
South of the Border Black Bean Burgers
(Bring La) Fiesta Roasted Sweet Potato Bowl
Everyday Lentil Lunch
Everything but the Kitchen Sink Potato Nachos

SALADS

Feeling Upbeet and Lively Lentil Salad

SOUPS/STEWS

Perfectly Spiced Spinach Lentil Soup

Butter Bean Me Up One-Pot Soup

Sweet and Savory Peanut Soup

Simple-to-Make Supergreen Mushroom and Potato Soup

Creamy Dreamy Arugula and White Bean Soup

Gourd-geous Nourishing Pumpkin Chili

Savory Vegan Gumbo with Okra

SIDES

Warm and Earthy Herbed Lentils

SNACKS

Crispy Miso Onion Chickpeas

CHAPTER 4

BERRIES

Out of all the foods in this great wide world, I've always had a special passion for berries. For me, growing up, these amazing treats were an introduction to the beauty, magic, and generosity of the natural world.

The first ones to ripen, sometime in June, were the little red thimbleberries. Next came the orange-pink salmonberries. Later in the summer, we would gorge ourselves (Okay, I would gorge myself) on stands of wild blackberries, raspberries, blueberries, and salal berries.

I have a memory, from around age three, of going with my friends to a blackberry patch and stuffing berry after berry into my purple mouth, practically vibrating with bliss as the beneficiary of such luscious abundance.

Our ancestors were hunter-gatherers, or more likely, gatherer-hunters. There's something deep and primal about ranging through the woods on the lookout for ripe berries. Foraging came naturally to my young self, and it still feels like one of the most authentically human things I do.

Berries can inspire us to consider that life is about more than survival. While much of homesteading is focused on growing enough to get by, foraging for berries in season reminds us that sometimes the human experience includes overwhelming bounty. Those sweet, juicy berries tell us that we're not here just to pay the rent, but to love our lives.

Growing up, I figured that anything so delicious that grows so wild and plentiful without needing human labor to sustain it must be proof of benevolent divinity. And once I discovered that berries are the healthiest of fruit, and among the healthiest of all

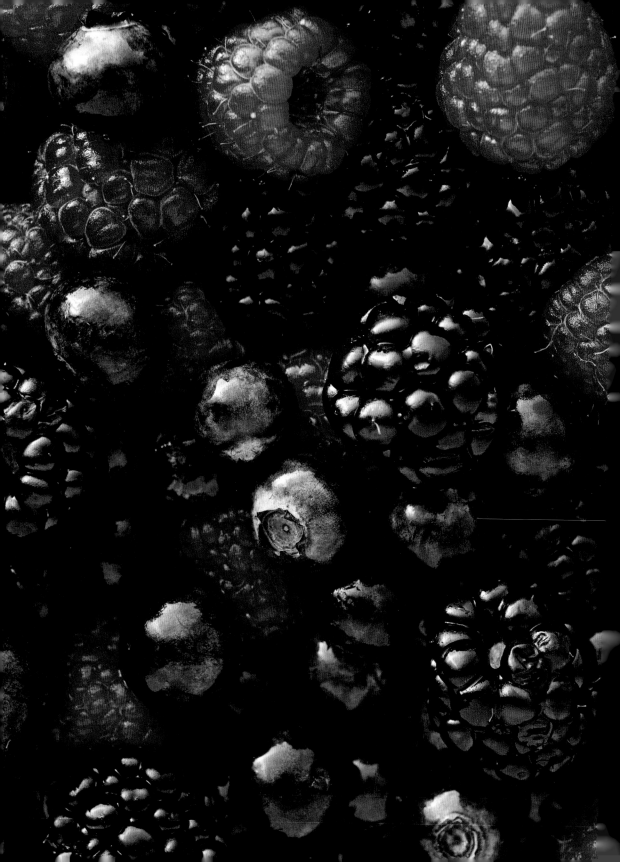

foods, I was even more impressed by the workings of the universe.

You might be surprised that I've included berries in this book on everyday superfoods. Sure, if you live in a part of the world where berries grow, and you can plant some or locate some wild stands, you can enjoy copious berries for free while they're in season.

But buying berries at the store or farmers market—even common domesticated varieties of blackberries, blueberries, strawberries, and raspberries—can be very expensive. And certain berries are already marketed as superfoods—the expensive kind. For example, acai berries, often dried or even powdered, command a premium price in upscale grocery stores and natural foods stores, and as ingredients in acai bowls and smoothies.

The good news is frozen berries can retain just about all their flavor and nutritional power and are generally much less expensive than fresh ones, providing a means to enjoy berries year-round.

Berry Nutrition Facts

Berries come in many different intense colors, each of which signals the presence of a different phytochemical or antioxidant that confers a host of health benefits. Don't worry if you can't access thimbleberries or other wild varieties; regular old raspberries, blueberries, and blackberries are among the foods that contain the highest antioxidant

FUN FACTS ABOUT BERRIES

Did you know that on April 28 each year, the United States celebrates the humble blueberry with National Blueberry Pie Day? They also celebrate National Blueberry Muffin Day on July 11—so many tasty ways to celebrate and enjoy blueberries!

capacity.[1] Other popular and potent berries include strawberries and cranberries. And depending on where you live, you may be able to find locally grown gooseberries, mulberries, and boysenberries.

Dark blue and red berries contain copious concentrations of anthocyanins, polyphenols, and antioxidants such as resveratrol. Berries of all hues tend to be high in vitamin C, vitamin K1, and manganese. And they're also a good source of fiber, with raspberries doing particularly well in that domain.

Why Berries Deserve Superfood Status

All those nutrients give berries disease-fighting and anti-inflammatory superpowers. For one thing, berries can improve your mood—and not just because they're fun to pick and delicious to eat. It turns out that some of the flavonoids in blueberries have been shown to decrease symptoms of depression in children and young adults.[2] In one study, researchers delivered blueberries in drink form so that they could offer identical-seeming placebos to a control group. The real blueberry group experienced marked improvement in mood.

Berries help the brain in the long term as well, aiding in protection against dementia, Parkinson's disease, and cognitive decline. In 2012, researchers from Harvard found that women who consumed at least one serving of blueberries or two servings of strawberries per week showed substantially slower rates of cognitive decline than those who abstained from berries.[3] A 2019 study by Rush University replicated this result, finding that those older people who ate the most strawberries had a 24 percent lower risk of developing Alzheimer's.

Another study[4] analyzed data from 16,000 women with an average age of 74. Those with the highest levels of blueberry consumption delayed their cognitive aging by as much as two and a half years. Biochemists surmise that, at least in part, it's the anthocyanidins and total flavonoids that give berries their brain-protecting powers.

The flavonoid nutrients in blueberries have also been shown to protect against the development of Parkinson's. Researchers' current best guess is that these compounds can cross the blood-brain barrier and prevent certain proteins from "clumping"—a phenomenon at the root of not just Parkinson's, but Alzheimer's, Creutzfeldt-Jakob, mad cow, and Huntington's diseases as well.[5]

Berries appear to be cancer-fighters, too. They've long been suspected as anti-cancer agents because of their impressive antioxidant profiles. Recent research credits their ability to boost the immune system, where there have been signs that they can help prevent or at least delay the progression of cancer.[6] A number of test-tube and animal studies have found that black raspberries may prevent mouth, colon, skin, and esophageal cancer, as well as certain breast cancers.[7]

Berries appear to bolster protection against cardiovascular disease as well. Population studies show a clear association between eating berries and avoiding heart disease; both in Finland and Iowa, those who ate the most berries, including strawberries, had the lowest risk of dying from a cardiovascular condition.[8] One way they may help is by helping to control cholesterol and blood pressure, two major risk factors for cardiovascular disease.

Berries don't just help you live longer—they might help you look better, too. It turns out, they can help protect your skin from free radical damage (again, those amazingly abundant antioxidants at work) and even acne. Blueberries and cranberries are particularly rich sources of resveratrol, which can inhibit the growth of the bacteria associated with acne.[9]

All the prebiotic fiber in berries serves as a yummy meal for the beneficial bacteria in your gut. And when those critters are thriving, your gut and all the systems that depend on them have the best chance of being healthy and strong.

Culinary Uses for Berries

Berries make one of the best snacks ever. Whether you're enjoying a refined handful arranged daintily on a plate, gorging yourself at a U-pick berry farm, adding frozen berries to a smoothie, or foraging from a wild patch, the sweetness, juiciness, and just-right texture of berries can really hit the spot. They also make a great dessert, either on their own or as part of a fruit salad or compote.

Berries, whether fresh or frozen, can also liven up oatmeal. A pro tip when you're in a hurry is to cook the oatmeal until it's done, and then cool it down with frozen berries. In just a minute, your oatmeal is cool enough to enjoy without burning your tongue and the berries are thawed through. Fresh and defrosted berries can also make delicious salad toppings.

Berries can also add some sweetness—or in the case of cranberries, tartness—to savory dishes. You can blend them into smoothies and smoothie bowls (especially the deep purple and black varieties, which add amazing color to the mixtures), and freeze them into popsicles. Berry

sauces can be used as salad dressings and dessert toppings.

To get the most nutrition out of your berries, here are a couple of tips. First, eat them raw whenever possible to preserve their flavonoids and antioxidants. And second, avoid consuming them with dairy, which can reduce your body's ability to absorb their polyphenols, the compounds largely responsible for their antioxidant activity.

FUN FACTS ABOUT BERRIES

Did you know that strawberries have a high concentration of a compound known as salicylates, which is the same ingredient found in aspirin? Next time you have a headache, try snacking on a few juicy strawberries to help relieve the pain. Strawberries aren't the only ones: blackberries, blueberries, and cranberries round out the list of berries rich in salicylates!

BERRY	PHYTONUTRIENT(S)	ANTIOXIDANT CAPACITY (TOTAL CONCENTRATION PER 100G)
Blueberries	Anthocyanins Ellagic Acid Tannins Ellagitannins Quercetin Gallic Acid Vitamin C (ascorbic acid) Resveratrol	525 mg/100 g
Blackberries	Anthocyanins Ellagic Acid Tannins Ellagitannins Quercetin Gallic Acid Vitamin C (ascorbic acid)	248 mg/100 g
Cranberries	Flavonols Phenolic acids Vitamin C (ascorbic acid)	120-315 mg/100 g
Raspberries	Anthocyanins Ellagitannins Hydroxycinnamic Acid Quercetin Vitamin C (ascorbic acid)	126 mg/100 g
Strawberries	Anthocyanins Ellagic Acid Gallic Acid Quercetin Vitamin C (ascorbic acid)	225 mg/100 g

BERRIES RECIPES

BREAKFAST

Hearty Blueberry Walnut Hotcakes

Warm Banana Chia Breakfast Pudding

SALADS

Minty Fresh Strawberry Salad

DESSERTS

Bright and Fruity Blueberry Lemon Bars

Summertime Strawberry Rhubarb Crisp

Velvety Chocolate Berry Dessert Cups

DRINKS

Purple Paradise Smoothie

Hemp-tastic Strawberry Shortcake Smoothie

CHAPTER 5

ALLIUMS

Once upon a time, according to an old Jewish folktale, a man heard from a traveler about a wealthy kingdom that didn't use onions in its cuisine. In fact, people there had never seen or heard of the tasty bulbs.

The enterprising man packed a cart with onions and traveled to the kingdom. And when he arrived, he presented the onions to the king.

The king loved them. And he rewarded the man by filling his cart with gold. Upon his return to his own village, the man told his neighbors what had happened. One of them reasoned that he could make even more money by introducing garlic to this kingdom. After all, garlic is even more pungent and delicious than onions!

The neighbor's intuition proved correct. The king adored garlic and proclaimed it the best-tasting food he had ever eaten.

Mere gold wouldn't adequately compensate for this delicacy. Instead, he sent the man home with the greatest treasure his kingdom could supply: a cart full of onions!

This story tells us a lot about the human love of alliums, a unique family of plants that are widely used in both everyday cooking and traditional medicine.

What Are Alliums?

Even if you haven't heard the term "allium" before, you're probably more familiar with these vegetables than you think. And you probably eat the most common ones, onions and garlic, pretty often. Other members of the family include shallots, leeks, chives, and scallions (also called green onions).

When I was a kid, onions and garlic served double duty. Not only did they

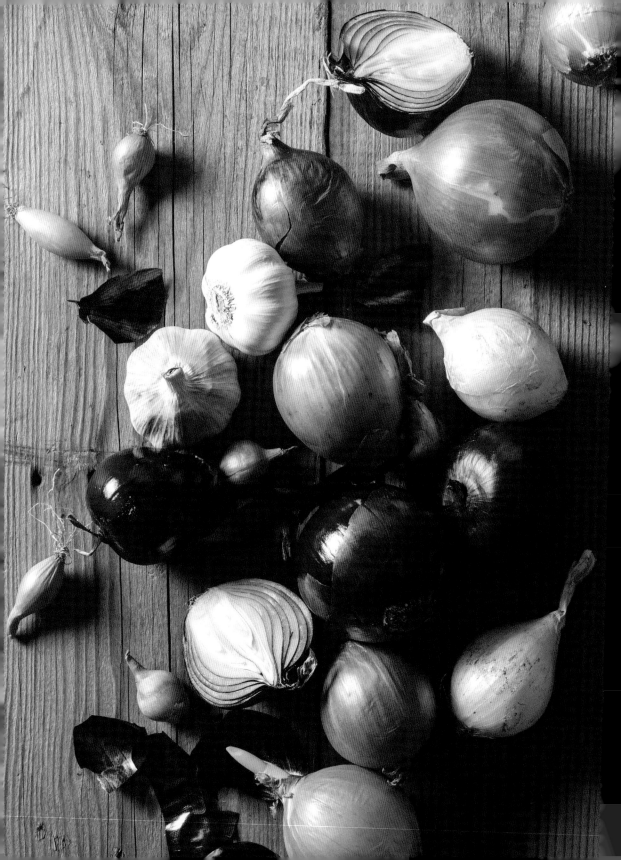

impart flavor to many of our meals, but they were a garden staple because of their ability to repel pests. We dotted them throughout our garden beds and at the ends of most rows, since the critters that would munch on our crops didn't enjoy garlic breath any more than lovers do. We left a lot of them in the ground and pulled them out as needed—you can't get much fresher than that!

Another nice thing about gardening with alliums is how forgiving they are of nutrient-poor and otherwise challenging soil, as well as a wide range of climates and ecosystems. As long as they get enough water, and not too much, they seem to be able to deal with a lot of limitations that would doom other garden plants. In fact, the one nutrient they need in order to produce that distinctive powerful odor that you smell when you cut them is sulfur, which fortunately, is found pretty much everywhere,[1] including in rocks, water, air, plants, and animals (including us).

If you've cooked with onions, you know how dramatically they can transform when cooked. Raw, they're sharp and spicy; cooked, they become quite tame. A small amount of crunchy raw onion can spice up a sandwich, but you don't want to go overboard. Cooked, though, that same onion becomes soft, succulent, and sweet.

Viewed in this way, alliums can help us set boundaries. They let us know that while it's good to be sweet and tender, sometimes it's appropriate to become feisty and even a bit cranky. They teach us to balance accommodation and assertiveness—yes and no.

And as we'll see, they contain amazing healing properties.

Allium Nutrition Facts

While the different members of the allium family have fairly similar nutritional profiles, I'm going to focus on the two most commonly used ones, onions and garlic. But you can expect roughly similar benefits from their cousins: leeks, shallots, chives, and scallions.

The most exciting nutritional feature shared by alliums is their remarkable antioxidant activity, which is delivered largely through powerful organosulfur compounds. They also provide a variety of vitamins and minerals, including B vitamins, vitamin C, folate, potassium, selenium, and manganese. They're rich in soluble fibers called fructans, as well as inulin, and when you eat them, you increase your body's ability to absorb and use iron and zinc.

Why Alliums Deserve Superfood Status

In addition to all their other nutritional benefits, one of the things that makes alliums extra special is their organosulfur compounds. It turns out these are released in response to predation; that is, when some critter starts munching on them. Their ability to defend their boundaries against attack is part of what makes alliums so good for us.

Alliums Protect the Immune System

Alliums are able to neutralize pathogens that can get into your body and make you sick. Their antimicrobial properties support your immune system's mandate to protect you from infection. One compound found in garlic, allicin, has been shown[2] to be effective against multidrug-resistant strains of E. coli, Candida albicans, and human intestinal parasites and viruses. This is hugely important, since overuse of pharmaceutical antibiotics has led to a severe decline in their effectiveness.

And if you want to cut way down on the bacteria in your mouth, a mouthwash that contains garlic[3] will do the trick. Whether you want to use such a product before a big date is totally up to you.

Alliums Protect Your Heart

The sulfur compounds in onions and garlic help your body fight cardiovascular diseases through many different mechanisms. These chemicals appear to regulate blood pressure, prevent blood clots in arteries, and lower blood lipids such as triglycerides and cholesterol.[4]

How big an effect can this have? A 2017 study[5] looked at over 3,000 adults over six years and found that those who consistently ate more allium vegetables reduced their risk of cardiovascular disease by a stunning 64 percent.

Alliums Fight Cancer

The organosulfur compounds in alliums appear to protect against cancer in at least two different ways: one, by triggering apoptosis, a process by which cancerous cells basically commit suicide for the sake of the larger organism; and two, by blocking the function of certain molecules that help cancer cells to reproduce.[6] And there are multiple studies that show a relationship between eating onions and garlic and having lower rates of several cancers, including those of the intestines, esophagus, prostate, and breast.[7]

Anti-Inflammatory Alliums Slow Aging

Alliums, especially garlic, have been shown in test-tube research to slow the aging process by retarding and reversing inflammation.[8] Some researchers theorize that a unique organosulfur compound found in garlic, thiacremonone, may be particularly responsible for this effect.[9]

And onions get in on the anti-inflammatory action as well. They are good sources of quercetin, which has been shown to relieve pain and reduce swelling from rheumatoid arthritis and osteoarthritis.[10]

Alliums Promote Digestive Health

Those wonderful fructans and inulin feed the beneficial bacteria in your large intestines, which allow them to thrive and proliferate. This means they can crowd out harmful bacteria, as well as produce butyrate and other short-chain fatty acids that your body needs to function optimally.

That said, if your gut microbiome is lacking in certain beneficial bacteria, then suddenly adding a lot of alliums to your diet can cause some digestive distress. The central culprit is probably the fructans, which provide the first letter of the acronym FODMAPs: a group of short-chain carbohydrates that we can handle only with sufficient microbiome support. For most people, the best solution isn't to eliminate FODMAPs forever, but rather to work with a gastroenterologist or dietitian to build up your gut "muscle" to put those FODMAPs to work for you.

How to Prepare and Serve Alliums

As we've seen, raw and cooked alliums have very different culinary properties. If you can, it's great to include both approaches in your diet on a regular basis. (There's some evidence that they have different health benefits depending on whether they're cooked or not.)

Because they're so pungent, allium serving sizes can be smaller than other vegetables. You can use them as spices or

FUN FACTS ABOUT ALLIUMS

Did you know that elephant garlic isn't actually garlic but a close relative to a leek? Even so, it has the same growth habit and bulbing process as traditional garlic varieties.

condiments rather than in full portions. So a recipe may call for one to two cloves of garlic (I like to double or triple the amount, just for fun), a half cup of chopped onion, and one medium leek or scallion. Of course, you can also feature onions or leeks as side dishes in their own right, and onion soup can highlight the sweet and yummy flavor of onions cooked to smooth and creamy perfection.

There are a couple of tricks that can help you get the most nutrition and flavor from alliums while avoiding the crying jags that sometimes accompany cutting onions.

To skip the tears, start with a sharp knife (and learn how to use it safely). You want to cut the onion without having to saw back and forth or put extra pressure on the blade, so it slices, rather than tears, the flesh. Some cooks remove the bulb of the onion by cutting out a conic section at the end that contains the root hairs and discarding it, but this seems like a waste to me. The National Onion Association, which

I assume to be an authoritative source on the matter, recommends[11] chilling the onion for half an hour before cutting. Some YouTube chefs suggest wetting a paper towel and holding it between your lips, as this is supposed to absorb the sulfurous gas that triggers the tears.

Or you can embrace the crying and play some of your favorite torch songs while you cook. (If you want to stick with the kitchen theme, try Sarah Vaughan's "Black Coffee." And if you have kids [or ever were one], you can't go wrong with "Cat's in the Cradle" by Harry Chapin.)

While the world debates the best ways to avoid ugly bawling while chopping onions, there's settled science on another front: how to get the maximum nutrition from your alliums. You'll get more of those wonderful organosulfur compounds if you take a nice juicy bite of a raw onion or chomp down on some raw garlic cloves than if you consume them cooked.

So you might think I'm advising you to eat all your alliums raw for optimal health. While you certainly can do that, there's an easier way to get all the nutritional goodness without going around with breath that scares away vampires. It turns out that if you cut an onion or garlic clove, it begins to release those compounds in response to the injury. If you wait 10 minutes or so before cooking, more of the antioxidants will survive the heat and remain bioavailable.

FUN FACTS ABOUT ALLIUMS

Did you know that elephant garlic can grow anywhere from 1 (0.454 kg) to 2 pounds (0.907 kg) in weight? According to Guinness World Records, the largest recorded weight for a bulb of elephant garlic was 2 pounds 10 oz (1.19kg).

Culinary Uses for Alliums

Just about any savory dish can be enhanced by the powerful flavors of cooked alliums.

Many dishes begin with a base of sautéed onions and/or garlic, or a variant like shallots or leeks. These include sauces, soups, and stews; stir-fries and scrambles; pasta dishes; and a variety of mains and sides from around the world. Cooked and raw alliums also add flavor to grain bowls and salads.

Garlic is most commonly grown in white, purple, and pink varieties.
Here are the most popular garlic varieties.
See the appendix for a complete list of garlic varieties
and their predominant flavors.

Hardneck (Allium sativum var. ophioscorodon)	Softneck (Allium sativum var. sativum)
In the hardneck family, there are eight subtypes of garlic: Purple Stripe, Marbled Purple Stripe, Asiatic, Glazed Purple Stripe, Creole, Turban, Rocambole, and Porcelain	In the softneck family, there are three subtypes of garlic: Artichoke, Middle Eastern, and Silverskin
Bogatyr: Marbled Purple Stripe Flavor: pungent and slightly spicy	**Nootka Rose:** Artichoke Flavor: rich and strong
Chesnok Red: Purple Stripe Flavor: distinctive long-lasting garlic flavor, great for roasting	**Rose du Lautrec:** Silverskin Flavor: subtle and slightly sweet
Music: Porcelain Flavor: sweet, pungent, hot when raw	**Rojo del Pais Baza:** Creole/Silverskin (dependent on growing conditions) Flavor: deep, long lasting
German Extra Hardy: Porcelain (most common variety in the United States) Flavor: mild, not hot or spicy	
Spanish Roja: Rocambole Flavor: pungent and complex flavor that is mildly hot when raw; when cooked the flavor is mellow and slightly sweeter	
Roja del Pais Baza: Creole/Silverskin (dependent on growing conditions) Flavor: deep, long lasting	

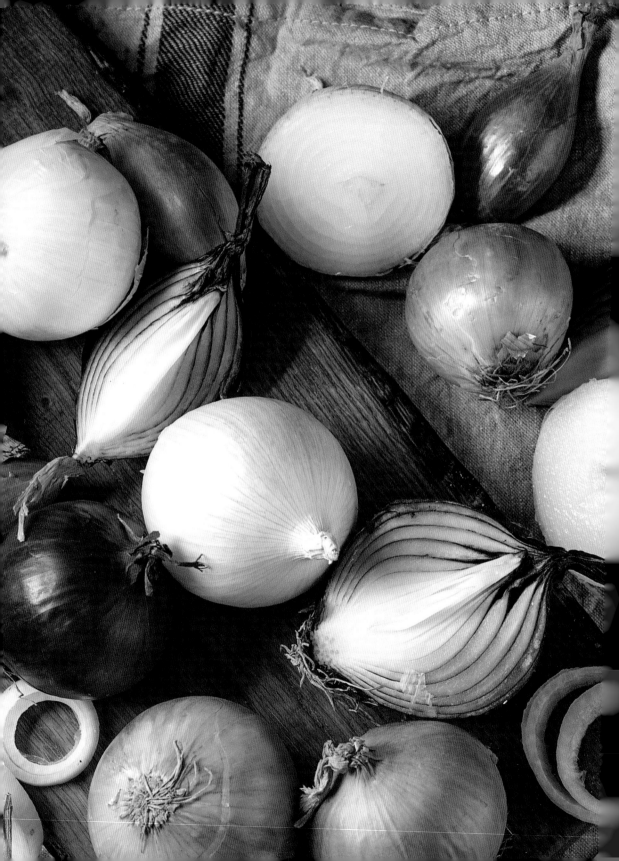

TYPE	FLAVOR	CULINARY USE
Chives	Delicate	Garnish: Bakes/Casseroles • Dips Potatoes • Soups
Leeks	Earthly, pungent, sweet	Greens: Used as flavor agent in homemade vegetable stock Whites: Bakes/Casseroles • Dressings Pasta • Sautés • Soups/Stews
Red Onion	Bright, pungent, sharp	Garnish: Stews • Pickled • Salads • Sandwiches/Wraps
Sweet Onion (Vidalia onion, Maui onion)	Mild, sweet	Caramelized • Onion Rings Soups/Stews • Sautés
Shallots	Pungent, garlicky, mildly sweet	Raw: Marinades • Salads • Vinaigrettes Cooked: Bakes/Casseroles • Soups/Stews Sauces • Sautés • Quiches
Scallions (green onions/spring onions)	Bright, fresh, savory	Whites and Greens: Sautés • Quick breads Raw as a garnish: Dips • Dressings Noodles/Pasta • Rice dishes Salads • Soups/Stews • Stir-fries
Yellow Globe Onion (Spanish onion)	Not too sweet and not too sharp	Bakes/Casseroles Caramelized • Curries Mirepoix • Soffritto Holy Trinity • Stir-fries Sauces • Soups/Stews • Rice Dishes

ALLIUMS RECIPES

BREAKFAST

Rockin' Rollup Lentil Sausage Breakfast Wraps
Easy Peasy Tofu Breakfast Bites
No Muss, No Fuss Breakfast Burrito
Harvest Grain Breakfast Bowl
Comforting Cauliflower Lentil Kitchari

MAINS

Simple Tri-Color Umami Stir-Fry
Plant-tastic Mushroom Ziti Bake
Built to Grill Beany Mushroom Burgers
Aromatic Veggie-Stuffed Acorn Squash
Mighty Greens Power Bowl
Pile 'Em High Black Bean Tostadas
Nice 'n' Cheesy Comforting Casserole
South of the Border Black Bean Burgers
Sprout and Flourish Grain Bowl
(Bring La) Fiesta Roasted Sweet Potato Bowl
Everyday Lentil Lunch
Kickin' Kimchi "Fried" Rice and Veggies
Vegged-Out Tofu Pad Thai
Everything but the Kitchen Sink Potato Nachos

SALADS

Fill Me with Warmth Tempeh and Kale Salad

Lemony Basil Farro Salad

Feeling Upbeet and Lively Lentil Salad

SOUPS/STEWS

Perfectly Spiced Spinach Lentil Soup

Butter Bean Me Up One-Pot Soup

Sweet and Savory Peanut Soup

Simple-to-Make Supergreen Mushroom and Potato Soup

Creamy Dreamy Arugula and White Bean Soup

Gourd-geous Nourishing Pumpkin Chili

Savory Vegan Gumbo with Okra

SIDES

Slow-Cooked Rainbow Collards

Herbaceous Wild Rice and Mushroom Stuffing

Warm and Earthy Herbed Lentils

SNACKS

Crispy Miso Onion Chickpeas

DRINKS

Fuel the Fire Cider

CHAPTER 6

HERBS AND SPICES

You know why it can be so hard for people to choose healthy foods? It's because unhealthy processed food is engineered to taste so good. Packed with excess salt, sugar, artificial additives, and unhealthy and often unnatural fats, these hyper-palatable, manufactured food products can overwhelm our taste buds and make fresh, healthy meals seem bland and boring by comparison.

Fortunately, you don't have to choose between tasty and healthy; food can be both. And the most powerful allies in your quest to create dishes that are both delicious and nutritious are ones that are most often overlooked in discussions of healthy foods: fresh and dried herbs and spices.

Humans have used herbs and spices to add flavor to their foods for a long time. Every culture around the world has its own unique spice blends, mixes, or associated culinary herbs. Think Herbs de Provence in France, the staggering variety of Indian masalas and curries, or Ethiopian berbere (which means "hot" in Amharic). Pick a country or region, and you'll find a distinctive flavor profile that comes from local herbs and spices.

Herbs and spices have also been used medicinally for just as long. And now science is, in many instances, confirming and providing mechanisms of action for traditional healers' uses of cinnamon, ginger, peppermint, black pepper, sage, and literally dozens of others. It turns out that not only are many herbs and spices delicious and aromatic, but they're also some of the healthiest foods ever studied.

When I was a kid, herbs and spices were how we took our simple meals from blah to wonderful. It was delightful to me—and still is—how just a teaspoon of cumin or

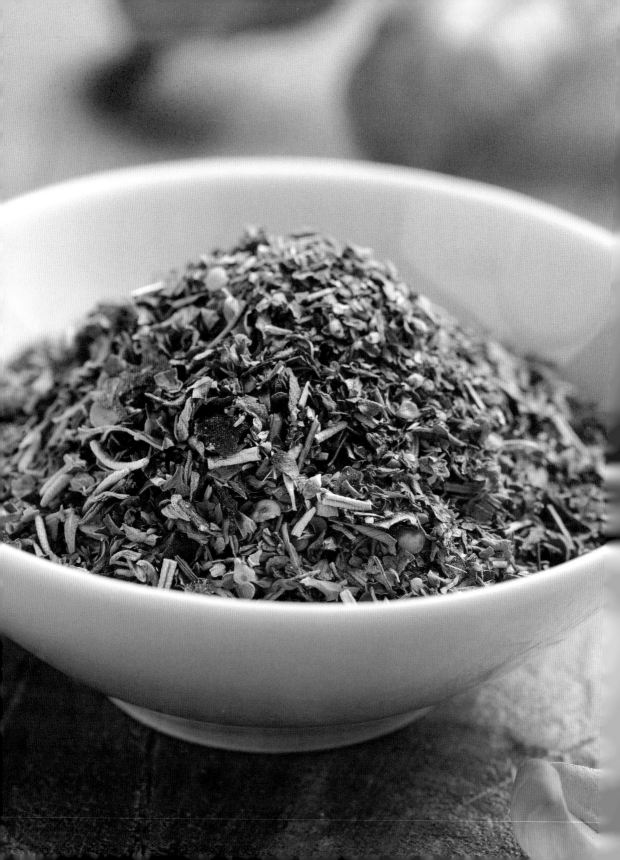

oregano could transform a dish from pedestrian to amazing. We celebrated how such a small amount of such an inexpensive ingredient could work so much magic.

If you've struggled to replace the sugary, salty, and fatty foods that make up so much of the standard modern diet, herbs and spices will soon be your new best friends. Knowing how to use them—which ones, how much, and how and when to add them to dishes—is what separates a workaday cook from a true chef.

But don't worry: cooking with herbs and spices isn't rocket science. Start by drawing upon the culinary traditions and cuisines you already enjoy: Mexican, Italian, Korean, South Indian, Thai, Cantonese, and so on. Then engage in bold experimentation. Use more than you might think, and try a lot of different combinations. Test the boundaries of sweet and savory, for example, by adding cinnamon, nutmeg, and allspice into a stir-fry or pasta sauce. Sprinkle some chili powder into your hot chocolate.

Notice the effect different spices have on you at different times of the year. In parts of the world with very hot summers, spicy foods are popular for a couple of reasons. First, spices keep food from spoiling. Second, eating them makes you sweat, which is your body's way of cooling down. (Which makes it very nice that "hot" spices tend to come from hot climates.)

There's a saying: Variety is the spice of life. Well, I'd argue that herbs and spices are the original spice of life. If you want more variety and intensity and joy in your life, start making friends with herbs and spices.

What Are Herbs and Spices?

Spices are generally the aromatic seeds, bark, flowers, and roots of plants, often those that grow in tropical regions. Herbs are generally from herbaceous plants (ones that lack woody stems), although some, like rosemary or bay leaf, do come from woody plants. Basically, herbs are leaves, and spices aren't.

The most common spices you'll find in any supermarket include black pepper, cinnamon, paprika, garlic powder and onion powder (alliums in the house!), powdered ginger, cloves, cumin, ground chili peppers, turmeric, and cardamom.

Common cooking herbs include parsley, basil, thyme, cilantro, dill, oregano, rosemary, mint, and sage. You can often find these in fresh form, sometimes even still growing in small pots of soil. But don't worry if you can't access fresh herbs; the dried forms are typically just as healthy, and actually more potent than when they're fresh, due to the concentration of flavors that occurs when the water is removed.

Herbs and Spices Nutrition Facts

Since there are hundreds of different herbs and spices, I have to generalize about their nutritional profiles. So the first generalization is that they're typically very high in antioxidants, which account for much of their disease-fighting properties. Chili peppers are an excellent source of antioxidants, vitamin C, carotenoids, and flavonoids.[1] Leafy greens such as parsley, cilantro, and basil contain high concentrations of vitamins A, C, and K.[2] Cumin is rich in minerals like iron, magnesium, calcium, and manganese, and even contains some omega-3 fatty acids.

Like many superheroes, spices can sometimes bring out the best in each other. An example is the way black pepper and turmeric work together. Turmeric has an impressive nutritional résumé, thanks largely to its main compound, the antioxidant and anti-inflammatory polyphenol curcumin. But there's a problem: our bodies don't easily absorb curcumin, so the amount of turmeric we'd need to eat to get the full benefit can be quite daunting. But adding black pepper to your turmeric-spiced dishes increases the bioavailability of curcumin by as much as a whopping 2,000 percent.[3]

Why Herbs and Spices Deserve Superfood Status

I'll share some of what we know about individual herbs and spices, but I don't want those facts to obscure the big point here: variety is key. Instead of focusing on just a couple of these powdered, flaked, or granulated superfoods, try to get as many into your diet as possible—even the ones I don't mention by name. They're basically all amazing!

Many herbs and spices are known to calm the GI tract, aiding digestion, alleviating constipation, and soothing an upset stomach. Peppermint has been shown to reduce symptoms of IBS.[4] Ginger contains compounds that reduce nausea and vomiting.[5] Cumin seeds can stimulate the production of bile, which helps digest fats.[6] Fennel seeds target bacteria that can cause indigestion.[7] Coriander seeds can speed up a sluggish digestive system.[8]

Herbs and spices are also potent helpers in the prevention of cancer. Sage, for example, can help block carcinogenic tumor formation by depriving tumors of blood.[9] An active ingredient in parsley, apigenin, also aids in preventing tumors from forming and lowering the growth rate of dangerous cancerous cells.[10]

Herbs and spices can also help keep blood pressure at a safe level and protect your heart. Chili peppers have been shown to help lower the risk of cardiovascular disease, largely due to their anti-inflammatory and antioxidant effects.[11] Cumin may aid heart health by targeting specific risk factors, including obesity and high LDL cholesterol.[12] Ginger can help reduce blood pressure, lowering the risk of both hypertension and heart disease.[13]

Many herbs and spices help the immune system do its job of keeping harmful pathogens at bay. Plants often use strong odors and tastes to repel predation, so it's no surprise that the herbs and spices best suited for adding flavor to food also exhibit antimicrobial properties. These include cilantro, mint, and one of the true antifungal and antibacterial superstars, cumin.

Cinnamon can help prevent and manage diabetes by decreasing sugar and fat levels in the blood. Chili peppers can also help decrease the risk of diabetes through their anti-inflammatory actions.[14] And ginger has been shown to lower A1c levels in type 2 diabetics, without the side effects of blood sugar–lowering medications.[15]

Herbs and spices can also help relieve pain. Ginger has been shown to be an effective treatment for migraines and menstrual cramps. Sage is a traditional pain remedy. Turmeric has been shown to be as effective as ibuprofen in reducing knee pain, without the drug's most common side effect, abdominal discomfort.[16]

Buying and Storing Herbs and Spices

Dried herbs and spices are more concentrated and potent than their fresh counterparts. A chef's rule of thumb is that if you substitute fresh herbs or spices for dried, triple the amount. For example, one teaspoon of dried oregano equals one tablespoon of fresh.

Dried herbs and spices last much longer than fresh ones and typically come powdered, as in garlic, onion, ginger, and cinnamon, or in small pieces (oregano, basil, thyme, and rosemary, for example). You can also get whole spices: cinnamon sticks, vanilla pods, nutmeg nuts, cumin and coriander seeds, and the like. While pre-ground spices are more convenient, buying them whole and grinding them yourself as needed will add even more flavor to your dishes. Whole spices also stay potent longer than ground ones.

Store dried herbs and spices in airtight containers, preferably made of glass. Keep the jars away from sunlight, which can degrade their potency. Instead, store them in a cool, dark, dry place like a pantry, kitchen cabinet (though not right above your stovetop), or drawer.

For dishes that call for spice blends, you can buy them premade or start with the ingredients and mix your own according to your preferences. You can find, for example, thousands of Indian garam masala recipes online, each with a different ratio of cinnamon to coriander to cardamom to cloves to cumin to chilis.

Fresh herbs may be "fresher," but unless you use them up quickly or store them properly, they can go to waste. It can be demoralizing to buy delicious-smelling sprigs of fresh dill or rosemary at an upscale market, take them home, and have to toss them, unused, a few days later.

Fresh herbs can, however, be among the most satisfying plants to grow. It doesn't take much space to have a little patch of basil, oregano, parsley, or other fresh herbs that you can harvest right at mealtime to add an extra-special freshness.

Fresh herbs work well in raw dishes, such as salads, or as garnishes for cooked dishes. They don't typically hold up in cooked dishes because 10 to 15 minutes of heat will cook away all the volatile oils and esters that give the fresh herbs their fresh flavor. If you use fresh herbs in a cooked dish, therefore, add them at the end to preserve that flavor.

Fresh root spices, like ginger, turmeric, and garlic, are best stored on a counter or in a cool dark place until you're ready to cut them. Once cut, place them in a breathable (not airtight) bag and store them in your refrigerator's crisper drawer. You can also peel and freeze ginger root. Scrape off the peel with a vegetable peeler, knife, or edge of a teaspoon, and cut the roots into smaller portions for use in recipes. I like to have a variety of teaspoon- and tablespoon-sized chunks in the freezer for stir fries, sauces, and dips. And the great thing about frozen ginger is that it grates easily and doesn't produce the "strings" you'll get when you grate fresh ginger.

To store fresh herbs for maximal longevity, clip off the bottom of their stems, remove any wilted or brown leaves, and put them in a glass container with about an inch of water at the bottom, like you would flowers. (I think a vase full of basil says "I love you" better than long stem roses any day, and I'm pretty sure my wife would agree!)

Unlike that flower bouquet, store your fresh herbs in the fridge, and change the water every couple of days. Otherwise, you will start to experience the questionable aroma of "eau de swamp."

Culinary Uses for Herbs and Spices

Herbs and spices are a great way to add punch, variety, flavor, and aroma to your cooking. You can create dishes that are sweet, salty, spicy, or herbaceous. By experimenting with different flavor profiles, you can turn an ordinary dish into a gourmet feast. And at the same time as you're tickling your taste buds, you're also eliminating the need for excess sugar, oil, and salt, which will make your cooking a lot healthier. And as we've seen, fresh and dried herbs and spices offer their own tremendous health benefits as well.

You can use herbs and spices in pretty much any savory dish you can imagine: soups, stews, pastas, roasted veggies, stir-fries, wraps, pizzas, sandwich fillings, dips, sauces, salad dressings, and more.

And some herbs and spices will add pizzazz to sweet dishes like desserts, dessert sauces, and hot drinks.

BASIL MAY HELP TO PREVENT OR TREAT:

Acne	Gout
Cancer	Cardiovascular disease
High Cholesterol (total, LDL, and elevated triglycerides)	Inflammation
High Blood Sugar	Stress

BASIL IS DELICIOUS WITH:

Allspice	Marjoram
Black Pepper	Mint
Celery seed	Oregano
Garlic	Parsely
Ginger	Rosemary
Lemongrass	Sage
Saffron	Sun-dried tomato
Thyme	

Adapted from Aggarwal, B, and Yost, D. *Healing Spices: How to Use 50 Everyday and Exotic Spices to Boost Health and Beat Disease*. New York: Sterling; 2011.

HOW TO USE BASIL

Easy Peasy Tofu Breakfast Bites, pg 132
Plant-tastic Mushroom Ziti Bake, pg 150
Lemony Basil Farro Salad, pg 184
Hearty Wild Rice, Mushroom, and Baby Broccoli Salad, pg 186
Minty Fresh Strawberry Salad, pg 188
Perfectly Spiced Spinach Lentil Soup, pg 196
Creamy Dreamy Arugula and White Bean Soup, pg 204
Warm and Earthy Herbed Lentils, pg 220

CUMIN MAY HELP TO PREVENT OR TREAT:

Asthma	Eczema/Itching
Allergies	Cardiovascular Disease and High Blood Pressure
High Cholesterol (total, LDL, and elevated triglycerides)	Inflammation/Pain
Colitis Symptoms (irritable bowel disease)	Pain
Dermatitis	

CUMIN IS DELICIOUS WITH:

Cardamom	Nutmeg
Cinnamon	Pumpkin Seed
Cacao	Turmeric
Clove	Vanilla
Ginger	

Adapted from Aggarwal, B, and Yost, D. *Healing Spices: How to Use 50 Everyday and Exotic Spices to Boost Health and Beat Disease*. New York: Sterling; 2011.

HOW TO USE CUMIN

Comforting Cauliflower Lentil Kitchari, pg 142
Aromatic Veggie-Stuffed Acorn Squash, pg 154
Pile 'Em High Black Bean Tostadas, pg 158
South of the Border Black Bean Burger, pg 162
(Bring La) Fiesta Roasted Sweet Potato Bowl, pg 168
Everyday Lentil Lunch, pg 170
Everything but the Kitchen Sink Potato Nachos, pg 176
Sweet and Savory Peanut Soup, pg 200
Sunset Glow Root Veggie Soup with Toasted Sunflower Seeds, pg 206
Gourd-geous Nourishing Pumpkin Chili, pg 208

GINGER MAY HELP TO PREVENT OR TREAT:

Arthritis (osteo and rheumatoid)	Heartburn/Gastrointestinal Issues and Indigestion
Asthma	Migraine
Cancer	Nausea and Motion Sickness
High Cholesterol (total, LDL, and elevated triglycerides)	Stroke
Cardiovascular disease	

GINGER IS DELICIOUS WITH:

Cardamom	Cumin	Parsley
Chile	Curry leaf	Sesame
Cinnamon	Fennel Seed	Turmeric
Clove	Garlic	Tamarind
Coriander	Onion	Vanilla

Adapted from Aggarwal, B, and Yost, D. *Healing Spices: How to Use 50 Everyday and Exotic Spices to Boost Health and Beat Disease*. New York: Sterling; 2011.

HOW TO USE GINGER

Sweet Baked Apple Walnut Oatmeal, pg 138
Comforting Cauliflower Lentil Kitchari, pg 142
Simple Tri-Color Umami Stir-Fry, pg 148
Kickin' Kimchi "Fried" Rice and Veggies, pg 172
Fill Me with Warmth Tempeh and Kale Salad, pg 180
Sweet and Savory Peanut Soup, pg 200
Sweet Vitality Carrot Cake, pg 246
Golden Glow Lemonade, pg 250
Soul-Soothing Golden Milk, pg 254
Enchanting Masala Chai, pg 256
Fuel the Fire Cider, pg 260
Purple Paradise Smoothie, pg 263

OREGANO MAY HELP TO PREVENT OR TREAT:

Alzheimer's disease	Cardiovascular Disease and High Blood Pressure
Candida, systemic fungal infections and yeast infections	Parasitic Infections and Bacterial Infections
Cancer	Metabolic syndrome
High cholesterol (total, LDL, and elevated triglycerides)	Insulin Resistance
Colitis symptoms (Inflammatory Bowel Disease)	Thrush (oral candida)

OREGANO IS DELICIOUS WITH:

Basil	Marjoram	Sage
Bay Leaf	Parsley	Sun-dried tomato
Chili	Rosemary	Thyme
Cumin	Pumpkin Seed	
Garlic	Onion	

Adapted from Aggarwal, B, and Yost, D. *Healing Spices: How to Use 50 Everyday and Exotic Spices to Boost Health and Beat Disease*. New York: Sterling; 2011.

HOW TO USE OREGANO

Rockin' Rollup Lentil Sausage Breakfast Wraps, pg 128
Easy Peasy Tofu Breakfast Bites, pg 132
Plant-tastic Mushroom Ziti Bake, pg 150
Nice 'n' Cheesy Comforting Casserole, pg 160
South of the Border Black Bean Burgers, pg 162
Feeling Upbeet and Lively Lentil Salad, pg 190
Super Seed Autumn Salad with Tart Pomegranate Dressing, pg 192
Gourd-geous Nourishing Pumpkin Chili, pg 208
Savory Vegan Gumbo with Okra, pg 210

TURMERIC MAY HELP TO PREVENT OR TREAT:

Acne/Blemishes	Gout
Allergies	Cardiovascular Disease and High Blood Pressure
Alzheimer's Disease	Inflammation
Arthritis (osteo and rheumatoid)	Eczema/Itching Psoriasis
Asthma	Pain
High Cholesterol (total, LDL, and elevated triglycerides)	Liver Disease
High blood sugar	

TURMERIC IS DELICIOUS WITH:

Allspice	Coriander	Mustard Seed
Black Pepper	Cumin	Onion
Caraway	Fennel Seed	Sun-Dried Tomato
Cardamom	Garlic	
Cinnamon	Ginger	

Adapted from Aggarwal, B, and Yost, D. *Healing Spices: How to Use 50 Everyday and Exotic Spices to Boost Health and Beat Disease.* New York: Sterling; 2011.

HOW TO USE TURMERIC

Easy Peasy Tofu Breakfast Bites, pg 132	Sweet and Savory Peanut Soup, pg 200
No Muss, No Fuss Breakfast Burrito, pg 134	Sunset Glow Root Veggie Soup with Toasted Sunflower Seeds, pg 206
Comforting Cauliflower Lentil Kitchari, pg 142	Sweet Vitality Carrot Cake, pg 246
Aromatic Veggie-Stuffed Acorn Squash, pg 154	Golden Glow Lemonade, pg 250
Nice 'n' Cheesy Comforting Casserole, pg 160	Soul-Soothing Golden Milk, pg 254
Everyday Lentil Lunch, pg 170	Mindfulness Moment Matcha Tea, pg 258
Uncomplicated Crunchy Kale Slaw, pg 182	Fuel the Fire Cider, pg 260
Butter Bean Me Up One-Pot Soup, pg 198	

HERBS AND SPICES RECIPES

BREAKFAST

Rockin' Rollup Lentil Sausage Breakfast Wraps

Easy Peasy Tofu Breakfast Bites

No Muss, No Fuss Breakfast Burrito

Sweet and Spice and Everything Nice Breakfast Bowl

Sweet Baked Apple Walnut Oatmeal

Harvest Grain Breakfast Bowl

Comforting Cauliflower Lentil Kitchari

Warm Banana Chia Breakfast Pudding

MAINS

Plant-tastic Mushroom Ziti Bake

Built to Grill Beany Mushroom Burgers

Aromatic Veggie-Stuffed Acorn Squash

Pile 'Em High Black Bean Tostadas

Nice 'n' Cheesy Comforting Casserole

South of the Border Black Bean Burgers

(Bring La) Fiesta Roasted Sweet Potato Bowl

Everyday Lentil Lunch

Kickin' Kimchi "Fried" Rice and Veggies

Vegged-Out Tofu Pad Thai

Everything but the Kitchen Sink Potato Nachos

SALADS

Fill Me with Warmth Tempeh and Kale Salad

Uncomplicated Crunchy Kale Slaw

Lemony Basil Farro Salad

Hearty Wild Rice, Mushroom, and Baby Broccoli Salad

Minty Fresh Strawberry Salad

Feeling Upbeet and Lively Lentil Salad

SOUPS/STEWS

Perfectly Spiced Spinach Lentil Soup

Butter Bean Me Up One-Pot Soup

Sweet and Savory Peanut Soup

Simple-to-Make Supergreen Mushroom and Potato Soup

Creamy Dreamy Arugula and White Bean Soup

Sunset Glow Root Veggie Soup with Toasted Sunflower Seeds

Gourd-geous Nourishing Pumpkin Chili

Savory Vegan Gumbo with Okra

SIDES

Herbaceous Wild Rice and Mushroom Stuffing

Warm and Earthy Herbed Lentils

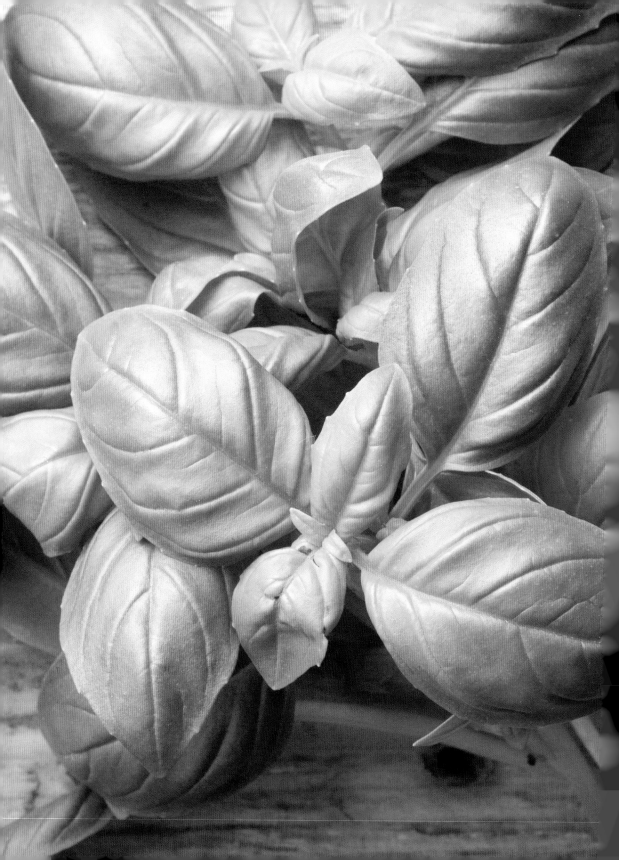

SNACKS

Zesty Chili Lime Kale Chips

Sweet and Savory Spiced Pecans

Super Seedy Granola

DESSERT

Sweet Vitality Carrot Cake

DRINKS

Golden Glow Lemonade

Cool as a Cucumber Matcha Refresher

Soul-Soothing Golden Milk

Enchanting Masala Chai

Mindfulness Moment Matcha Tea

Fuel the Fire Cider

Purple Paradise Smoothie

Hemp-tastic Strawberry Shortcake Smoothie

CHAPTER 7

SWEET POTATOES

As a kid, I had almost no experience with sugar or sugary foods. Berries were basically the closest thing I had to dessert. Of course, I didn't mind, because I didn't know what I was missing; heck, kale and turnips tasted darn good to me. But a few times a year, on really special occasions, we'd fire up the tiny stove in our log cabin (a treat in that British Columbia winter, I can tell you!) and bake up some sweet potatoes.

The smell by itself would make my mouth water—as does the memory of it as I type this. As the caramelizing sugars bubbled and dripped onto the foil layer that we placed on the oven floor, I could hardly contain my excitement. I looked forward to a baked sweet potato the way some people anticipate some ultrarich double chocolate cheesecake.

Despite everything I've learned about the health benefits of sweet potatoes—which we'll get to in a minute—there's still a part of my brain that believes anything that sweet has to be unhealthy. When I found out that they can actually stabilize blood sugar, and so can be good for people with type 2 diabetes, I was thunderstruck.

There's a saying in business that there are three essential qualities to every product and service—quality, speed, and price—and that you can have any two, but never all three. In other words, you can get good and fast, but you have to pay a lot for it. You can get fast and cheap but at the expense of quality. And so on. Those companies that figure out how to create good, fast, and inexpensive offerings are exceedingly rare.

In the world of food, the two qualities that usually involve trade-offs, at least in many people's minds, are taste and health.

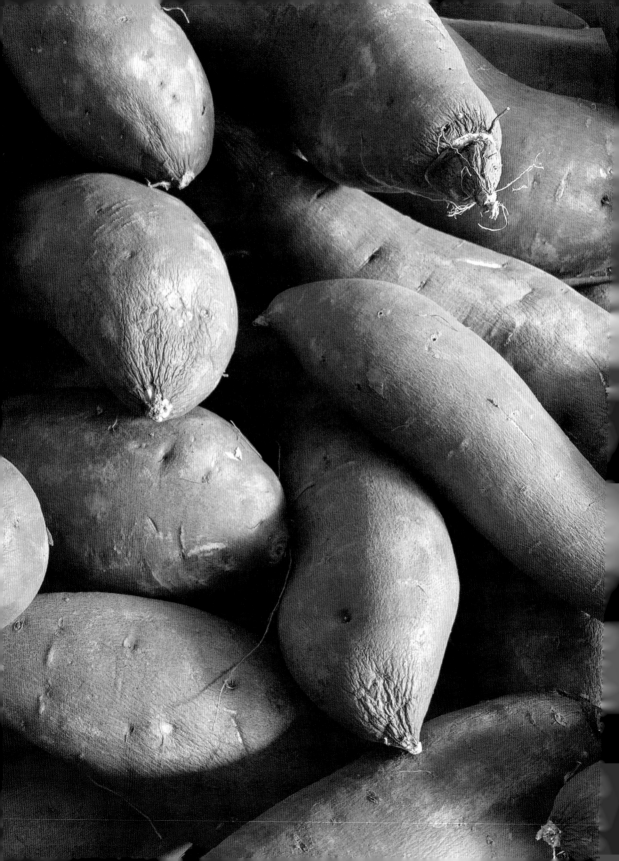

"Health food" is bland at best. And delicious food is bad for you and probably fattening. It's not true, of course—I'd argue that health-promoting foods can be utterly delectable if you know how to prepare them. But there's no denying that, say, dandelion greens won't light up your taste buds in quite the same way a doughnut will.

That said, whoever invented the sweet potato hit the jackpot: a superfood that tastes like a really sweet dessert. The different varieties check so many nutritional boxes—vitamins, antioxidants, fiber, vital minerals like copper and manganese—and taste so sweet and delicious!

In terms of names, I have to clear up a couple of misconceptions. First, sweet potatoes aren't the same as yams, even though marketers in the 1930s borrowed the word to describe unfamiliar orange-fleshed varieties and distinguish them from the white-toned sweet potatoes people were used to.[1]

Second, they aren't actually potatoes; they're not even in the same family. In terms of taste and texture, sweet potatoes are generally sweeter and juicier than regular old spuds.

So now that we know they aren't yams or potatoes, what exactly are sweet potatoes? Why are they so good for you? How can they support your health? And how can you get more of this amazing superfood into your diet?

What Are Sweet Potatoes?

The sweet potato, *Ipomoea batata*, is a root tuber, similar to beets, carrots, and turnips. A relative of morning glory or bindweed, it originated in tropical regions of Central and South America—or so has long been thought. While fossil evidence reveals the plant growing in the Americas 35 million years ago, scientists recently discovered fossilized morning glory leaves 12 million years older than that in what is now India.[2]

Regardless of its initial origin, the sweet potato quickly spread around the world, thanks to humans who prized its taste, nutritional profile, and ability to grow in varied conditions.

There are two main classes of sweet potato, firm and soft. The firm ones resemble true potatoes in how they cook, remaining firm and dry even when baked. The soft ones are so named because they soften considerably (and retain water) as they cook.

You may encounter only a few varieties of sweet potato in your local grocery store. The most common in the US is the Beauregard, with reddish-orange skin and deep-orange flesh. Similarly hued common varieties include garnet (the ones I enjoyed most as a child) and jewel.

You can often find white sweet potatoes, which have more crumbly flesh inside golden brown skin. They are milder tasting than the orange ones (and—full disclosure—deliver fewer antioxidants).

There are also stunning purple sweet potatoes, also called Okinawan sweet potatoes, which were imported to Japan from the Americas in the 16th century and have become a staple of the super-healthy Okinawan diet. This island is one of the "Blue Zone" areas of remarkable human health and longevity, and many residents credit their extended "healthspan"—the longest in the world—to daily consumption of these antioxidant-rich roots. Researchers have confirmed the association: traditionally, Okinawans have gotten over 60 percent of their calories from that single food.

If you think that's extreme, wait until you meet the Papua New Guinean Highlanders, who get 90 percent of their calories from sweet potatoes. And they also reap the health benefits: one study from 1994 found they rarely experienced heart disease, strokes, or indeed any other modern chronic diseases.[3]

These groups aren't outliers—many other cultures around the world have been relying on sweet potatoes for a long time. In fact, they may be one of the oldest foods known to humanity.

Sweet Potato Nutrition

Compared to white potatoes, sweet potatoes contain more vitamins and antioxidants. To get the most nutritional benefit from sweet potatoes, eat the skins, which may contain 10 times the antioxidant power of the flesh.

Sweet potatoes are high in beta-carotene, vitamin C, and several B vitamins, including pantothenic acid, niacin, and vitamin B6. The beta-carotene, which imparts an orange color, gets converted by your body into all-important vitamin A. A single sweet potato contains, on average, twice as much vitamin A as your body needs. And since it's in carotene form, your body can easily eliminate the excess, so there's no worry about vitamin A toxicity, which can happen when you get the vitamin from supplements or animal sources such as fish or cow's liver.

You can get beta-carotene, the most "famous" of the carotenoids, from whole plant foods like sweet potatoes and also in supplement form. But researchers found that isolating beta-carotene from its carotenoid cousins can cause imbalances that can severely compromise your health. One study of 29,000 Finnish smokers found that those who took supplemental beta-carotene had a much higher probability of developing lung cancer than those who got a placebo pill. A similar American study that included 18,000 smokers and asbestos workers also found an increased incidence of lung cancer in the beta-carotene group, as well as a 17 percent higher mortality rate.[4]

But when eaten in foods, where it is always accompanied by and in balance with

Carolina Ruby	Skin: Deep reddish purple Flesh: Dark orange
Covington	Skin: Rosy Flesh: Deep orange
Excel	Skin: Orange tan Flesh: Coppery orange
Jewel	Skin: Coppery Flesh: Bright orange
Okinawan	Skin: Purple Flesh: Light puple
Red Garnet	Skin: Reddish purple Flesh: Orange

an entire suite of carotenoids, it's been shown to have powerful health effects, especially in preventing cancer and enhancing vision (which we'll cover later.)

Sweet potatoes are also rich in fiber, including resistant starch, and are good sources of many essential minerals, including potassium, manganese, magnesium, iron, and copper. They also contain a modest but helpful amount of protein (about 4 grams per cup of cooked sweet potato). And purple sweet potatoes in particular are high in a potent family of antioxidants called anthocyanins.

Why Sweet Potatoes Deserve Superfood Status

The next time you look at a sweet potato (especially one of the orange or purple ones), I want you to picture a fully stocked pharmacy. Here are just a few of the health benefits of eating sweet potatoes on the regular.

Sweet Potatoes Support Digestive Health

Sweet potatoes, and particularly their skin, are an excellent source of fiber. Fiber is important for your digestive health, helping to prevent constipation and serious diseases such as colon cancer. Some of that fiber comes in the form of resistant starch, which is so named because it resists digestion in your small intestine.

Scientists used to think that this starch acted simply as a mechanical "broom" to keep things moving, but recent discoveries about the nature and function of the microbiome have changed that perspective. Now we know that resistant starch is food for the beneficial bacteria in your colon, which perform a whole host of functions essential for you to thrive.

Sweet Potatoes Support a Healthy Heart

Sweet potatoes are high in potassium, which works in balance with the sodium in your body to maintain healthy blood pressure. They're also high in copper, a metal essential for the production of red blood cells. Low levels of copper have been linked to several cardiovascular risk factors, including high LDL ("bad") cholesterol levels.

The high fiber content of sweet potatoes can also lower LDL cholesterol, which has been shown to be the most significant risk factor for heart disease.

Sweet Potatoes Help Stabilize Blood Sugar

The fiber and complex carbohydrates in sweet potatoes can help keep your blood sugar stable, which is important for preventing and managing diabetes. Several randomized clinical trials found that participants who added sweet potatoes to their diets lowered their A1c levels.[5] (A1c is a marker of how much sugar was in the blood over the prior three months.)

An added bonus of stable blood sugar is that it can support a healthy weight, since you don't experience the dips that tell your body to eat right now.

Sweet Potatoes Can Support Your Immunity

Sweet potatoes are rich in antioxidants that prevent free radical damage in your body. Just one cup of baked sweet potato gives you more than half your daily requirement of vitamin C, which helps with wound healing and tissue repair.

The high levels of beta-carotene in sweet potatoes help your body make immune cells that stave off infections and disease and have antitumor effects. Purple sweet potatoes in particular contain especially potent antioxidants called anthocyanins.

Sweet Potatoes Are Good for Your Eyes

Sweet potatoes contain several nutrients that have been linked to improved eye health and vision. Some of the most powerful are the carotenoids, including alpha-carotene, beta-carotene, lutein, and zeaxanthin.

Orange sweet potatoes (as well as other orange plants, including carrots) have particularly high concentrations of carotenoids.

It's not just the orange sweet potatoes that are good for your vision, though. A class of anthocyanins called PSPA, derived from purple sweet potato roots, might also benefit your eyes by encouraging the health and growth of retinal pigment epithelial (RPE) cells.

RPE cells help your eyes absorb light (which is kind of crucial to sight). They also trigger an immune response to any threat to eye health.

Sweet Potatoes Fuel Your Brain

Sweet potatoes also contain compounds like choline and manganese that your brain needs to function at its best. Choline is an essential nutrient for brain growth and development. You can also see it in the name of the neurotransmitter acetylcholine that sends messages between cells. Insufficient acetylcholine can impair cognition, memory, and even movement.[6]

Manganese is also important for brain health. It binds to neurotransmitters and helps move electrical impulses through your body faster.

The anthocyanins unique to purple sweet potatoes may also have memory-enhancing properties.

Sweet Potatoes Can Help Ease Stress and Anxiety

Sweet potatoes may help you relax. They're high in magnesium, which has been shown to play a role in calming the brain. Magnesium deficiency has been linked to depression, mood disturbances, and headaches.

Sweet Potatoes Can Help Boost Fertility

Sweet potatoes are excellent sources of vitamin A and iron, two nutrients essential for healthy reproduction.

Sweet Potatoes Can Help Fight Cancer

Sweet potatoes are a rich source of cancer-fighting antioxidants, especially in their skin. They have other anticancer properties, too.

Up to 80 percent of the protein in sweet potatoes is a type of storage protein known as sporamin. This unique protein appears to help inhibit several cancers, including those of the tongue, gallbladder, colon, and rectum. It has also been shown capable of slowing cancer cell growth and reducing cell migration and invasion in metastatic cancers.

Sweet potato peels, particularly those of the purple varieties, may be especially powerful when it comes to the prevention of cancers of the breast, colon, ovary, lung, and head/neck.

Fun fact about sporamin: it acts as a "defensive protein" in the sweet potato root and leaves, making the plant less yummy to predators. And sweet potato plants look out for each other; when one plant gets its leaves nibbled, it releases chemical signals that tell neighboring plants to produce more sporamin.[7]

Some agronomists are hoping to "borrow" sweet potatoes' genes and bioengineer them into other plants, such as cauliflower and tobacco, in the hopes that it will boost those crops' resistance to pests. Fortunately, you don't have to genetically modify yourself to get the immune benefit of sporamin; just eat sweet potatoes!

Sweet Potatoes Are Anti-Inflammatory

Eating sweet potatoes may also help reduce inflammation, a condition that's linked to pretty much every single chronic disease ever studied. In addition to the common inflammation fighters like beta-carotene, vitamin C, and magnesium, sweet potatoes' potent collection of antioxidants also plays a role here. One of the antioxidants that's found most abundantly in purple sweet potato flesh is called cyanidin, which may reduce inflammation specifically in the digestive tract.

How to Buy and Store Sweet Potatoes

Next time you shop for sweet potatoes, look for those with uniformly colored skin that isn't cracked or otherwise blemished. Give them a quick squeeze (or take your time; I won't judge) to make sure there's no squishiness that might indicate rotting.

Store sweet potatoes on your countertop or in a pantry; they like it cool and dry, but not refrigerated. Putting them in a wicker basket will encourage airflow that can keep them fresh longer. But don't let them sit for too long; depending on the temperature and humidity in your kitchen,

and how old they were when they arrived home, they should be good for up to a few weeks. If one starts to rot, get rid of it, as the gas it gives off can cause the others to begin breaking down as well.

How to Prepare and Serve Sweet Potatoes

Sweet potatoes are best eaten cooked. Raw sweet potatoes have an enzyme inhibitor that makes it hard for your body to digest the sporamin and other proteins. You can cook them in various ways: boiling, steaming, microwaving, baking whole, and baking or roasting cut pieces (like cubes, wedges, or rounds). One of my favorite methods is to cut them lengthwise and bake the halves face down on a tray lined with parchment paper. You can then use the halves as "boats" for various toppings—or just eat them straight away (I've definitely done that more than once!).

ORANGE SWEET POTATO	GOLDEN, RUSSET, WHITE POTATO	RED, PURPLE/BLUE POTATO
High in fiber	High in fiber	High in fiber
High in Vitamin A	Resistant starch (especially cooled, cooked potatoes)	Vitamin C
Antioxidants: Carotenoids Alpha-carotene Beta-carotene Lutein • Zeaxanthin	Vitamin C	Antioxidants: Anthocyanins Cyanidin
Vitamin C	Potassium	Potassium
Potassium	Magnesium	Maganese
Panthothenic acid (vitamin B5)	Vitamin B6	Magnesium
Vitamin B6	Phosphorus	Copper
Manganese	Niacin (vitamin B3)	Iron
Magnesium	Folate	Vitamin B6
Copper	Choline	Choline
Choline	4 grams of protein per cup	4 grams of protein per cup
4 grams of protein per cup		

Although sweet potatoes are not from the same botanical family as white and red/purple potato varieties, they do share a few nutrients in common. This table illustrates the similarities and differences between the tubers and spuds, and why we consider sweet potatoes to be super!

Culinary Uses for Sweet Potatoes

Oh, there are so many wonderful ways to add sweet potatoes to your life! In addition to topping baked sweet potatoes with black beans, guacamole, plant-based cheese, or sautéed onions and mushrooms, they make a great seasonal side dish—think about mashed sweet potatoes or the (misnamed) candied yams that graced many 20th-century American tables at Thanksgiving.

They also make a great nonseasonal side dish when coated in herbs and spices, baked in wedges, and served with a piquant or spicy dipping sauce—think really healthy french fries.

You can cook cubed or diced sweet potatoes in a stovetop skillet, maybe with onions and garlic (three cheers for alliums— see Chapter 5) as well as your favorite spices (hooray for spices—see Chapter 6). If you have a spiralizer, you can create sweet potato "zoodles" (or maybe "swoodles")

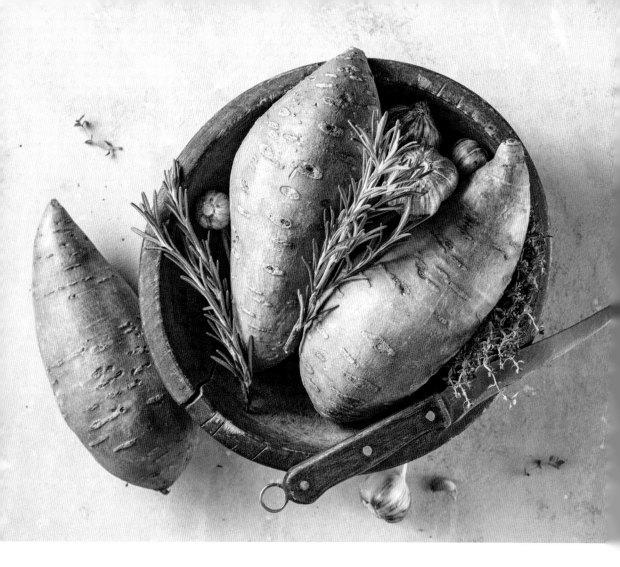

that you can then boil briefly to use as a base for your favorite pasta dishes.

Sweet potatoes can sweeten and add texture to chilis, stews, and casseroles. You can add diced and roasted sweet potatoes to grain bowls and breakfast scrambles. Diced or shredded, they can serve as the main ingredient in hashes.

And since they're so sweet, you can also use them in desserts, from sweet potato pies to healthy plant-based brownies to oil-free cakes. The simplest way to enjoy dessert sweet potatoes is to take some cooked purple ones, spread a bit of peanut butter on top, and then dust them with cacao powder. Close your eyes and you'll swear (or affirm, if you don't want to swear) that you're feasting on an ultra-decadent peanut butter brownie.

SWEET POTATO RECIPES

BREAKFAST

Sweet and Spice and Everything Nice Breakfast Bowl

MAINS

Pile 'Em High Black Bean Tostadas

(Bring La) Fiesta Roasted Sweet Potato Bowl

SOUPS/STEWS

Sweet and Savory Peanut Soup

Sunset Glow Root Veggie Soup with Toasted Sunflower Seeds

SIDES

Sublime Sweet Potato Mini Drop Biscuits

CHAPTER 8

NUTS AND SEEDS

 Nuts and seeds may be small, but they pack a major health and nutritional punch.

As a constantly moving and inquisitive little kid, I needed a lot of energy to get through the day. And between meals, my most common and beloved high-energy snack was trail mix. This wasn't some commercial trail mix that featured yogurt-covered pretzels and M&Ms. Mostly it consisted of roasted and salted nuts and seeds, with maybe a few raisins for sweetness.

After we moved to California when I was 10, we got most of our nuts directly from farmers markets and farm stands—including 10-pound bags of fresh walnuts in the shell. For the first time, I saw where nuts came from and discovered how much effort goes into getting the meat out of the shell. I could sit for an hour with a handheld nutcracker, feeding one walnut after another into its metal jaws and then into my mouth.

Around that age, I began to fancy myself a vegan chef, eager to show people that anything they could do with meat, I could do better with plants. And one of the most successful examples was my nut loaf, a meatloaf analogue that blended nuts, tofu, veggies, and spices into a hearty, tasty, and protein-rich meal.

Some people are surprised to hear that nuts and seeds are part of my healthy diet—thinking, no doubt, of pop-top cans or jars of nuts that are fried and coated in sugar and artificial flavorings. There's no question that flavoring and roasting nuts and seeds has the potential to downgrade their nutritional benefits, but the tradeoff is that they become more delicious and snackable,

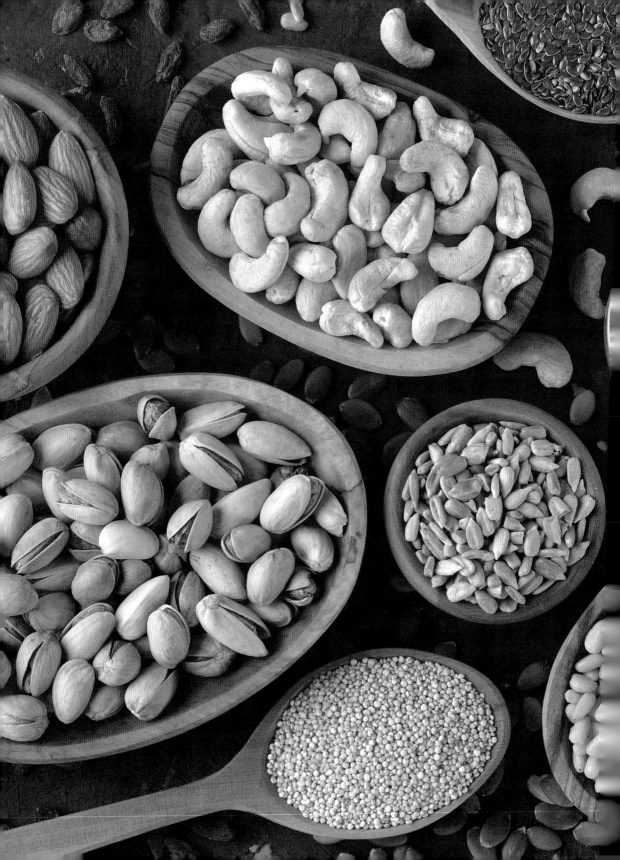

while still providing a good amount of nutritional benefits.

Relative to their caloric and nutritional density, even most flavored and salted nut products are not even that high in sodium, surprisingly enough. It turns out that when the salt is on the outside of a food—think mixed nuts or tortilla chips—a little goes a long way.

What makes nuts and seeds so powerful nutritionally? The way I think about it, they are the ultimate expression of life's potential to keep going. Each nut or seed literally has the instructions within it—the DNA—to build an entire tree or bush. And that new plant may produce tens of thousands or even millions of nuts or seeds, each of which contains the genetic information needed to make more plants, and so on and so on.

The abundance of nuts and seeds represents a calculated survival strategy for the plant. Since most will get eaten or end up on inhospitable ground, the plant overproduces like crazy to give itself the best odds to reproduce.

When you partake of that concentrated intelligence and abundance, you're consuming the creative force of life itself. And all the nutrients in the nut or seed that are needed to nurture a new life become available to you.

While science is just discovering many of the health benefits of nuts and seeds, it's not exactly news, as they've been staples of human diets for longer than most of us can even imagine. Archaeological remains from Israel of a meal that someone purportedly consumed around 780,000 years ago revealed that nuts were part of their diet.[1]

What Are Nuts and Seeds?

A seed is the mature fertilized ovule of a plant, consisting of three parts: an embryo, a food source, and a protective shell. A nut is a seed with a hard outer shell that doesn't open when the seed is mature. So all nuts are seeds; but not all seeds are nuts, because some lack that hard shell.

Things get more complicated from there. Sunflower seeds have a hard shell but are still seeds. Pine nuts are seeds, not nuts; peanuts are neither (remember them from the legumes chapter?). And technically peach pits are seeds (and maybe even nuts), but I don't recommend adding them to your trail mix or making them into peach pit butter.

Trying to figure it all out can make you feel a little nutty. So let's stick to common-sense categories and not worry too much about where a particular nut or seed belongs. With that strategy, here's a list of common nuts: pecans, walnuts, cashews, almonds, hazelnuts, Brazil nuts, macadamias, pistachios, pine nuts, and chestnuts. And here are some common seeds: sesame, sunflower, chia, flax, hemp, pumpkin, and poppy.

Nuts and Seeds Nutrition

Various nuts and seeds offer different nutritional benefits but have in common those related to the task of turning themselves into plants. They're all rich in high-quality plant proteins and fats, and are good sources of dietary fiber and B vitamins such as B6 and folate. Most nuts and seeds are full of minerals, including magnesium, iron, phosphorus, calcium, and zinc. And they contain powerfully protective antioxidants, such as tocopherols (basically, the vitamin E family) and phytosterols.

Some nuts and seeds are particularly rich in omega-3 fatty acids. Flaxseeds and chia seeds are all high in these anti-inflammatory fats that support brain function. In terms of antioxidant potential, the leaders are walnuts, pecans, and chestnuts.

And then there's the Brazil nut, which is the richest known source of dietary selenium, a trace mineral that's otherwise challenging to get on a plant-based diet. A single nut contains double your daily requirement.[2]

Why Nuts and Seeds Deserve Superfood Status

Like the other superfoods featured in this book, nuts and seeds aren't one-hit

wonders, addressing just a single disease or condition. Here's a (short) list of the health benefits of regular (moderate) consumption of these crunchy and tasty treats.

Nuts and Seeds May Help You Live Longer

In 2013, researchers pooled the results of the most ambitious health studies ever conducted: the Nurses' Health Study, which followed over 76,000 women from 1980 through 2010, and the Health Professionals Follow-Up Study, which assessed the health of over 42,000 men from 1986 through 2010. Each participant was asked about their nut consumption when they joined the study and then again every 2 to 4 years. While there were no doubt other factors involved (as there almost always are in observational studies), it's also a fact that those who ate one ounce of nuts at least seven times per week were 20 percent less likely to die during the course of the study than the nut avoiders.[3]

Another study found that the Seventh Day Adventists in Loma Linda, California, who ate nuts at least five times per week gained, on average, an extra two years of life expectancy.[4]

Nuts and Seeds May Prevent Heart Disease

You might not think that a group of relatively high-fat foods could help prevent heart disease, but nuts and seeds can do just

NUTS/SEEDS	SERVING	PROTEIN PER SERVING
Almonds	⅓ cup	7 grams
Brazil Nuts	6 kernels	4 grams
Cashew Nuts	⅓ cup	8 grams
Chia Seeds	2 tablespoons	4 grams
Flaxseeds	2 tablespoons	3 grams
Hemp Seeds	2 tablespoons	6 grams
Peanuts	⅓ cup	8 grams
Pumpkin Seeds	2 tablespoons	5 grams
Sesame Seeds	2 tablespoons	4 grams
Sunflower Seeds	2 tablespoons	4 grams
Walnuts	⅓ cup	5 grams

that—at least when eaten in moderation. Nuts have been shown to lower LDL cholesterol levels, decrease inflammation, prevent blood clots that might otherwise cause heart attacks and strokes, and lower blood pressure.[5]

In a 2021 Iranian study of 6,500 adults, those eating the most nuts had a lower risk of cardiovascular disease than those who consumed the least.[6] And Seventh Day Adventists who ate nuts at least five times a week cut their risk of heart disease in half.[7]

And let's not forget about the seeds. Flaxseeds in particular are extremely good for heart health. A 2015 study found that people with compromised arteries who ate flax meal while taking statins had lower total and "bad" LDL cholesterol than those who relied just upon the drug.[8] And some of the compounds in flax appear not just to help prevent and halt atherosclerosis, but may actually be able to contribute to reversing the process.[9]

Hemp seeds may also benefit your heart. Studies show they can help prevent arterial blockages by lowering cholesterol levels, protecting the heart after a cardiac event, and lowering high blood pressure, a major risk factor for heart disease.[10]

And chia seeds also get into the act, thanks in part to their rich concentrations of ALA, one of the omega-3 fatty acids. One 2014 randomized controlled trial found that chia flour lowered the blood pressure of people with preexisting hypertension.[11]

Nuts and Seeds Fight Cancer

Walnuts contain nutrients that can block the progression of prostate[12] and breast cancers.[13] Flaxseeds are also powerful cancer suppressors. In addition to their omega-3 fats, they contain a class of antioxidants called lignans, which have been studied for their ability to reduce the size, growth, and spread of breast cancer cells, as well as promote the death of those cells.[14]

There's reason to think that chia seeds can also help lower your risk of certain cancers. They're rich in ALA fatty acid, which has been shown to decrease the viability of both breast and cervical cancer cells.[15]

Nuts and Seeds May Prevent Type 2 Diabetes

Because nuts are high in fats and protein, they can help regulate blood sugar and prevent the kinds of spikes that occur with diabetes. Almonds in particular have been studied for their ability to positively impact blood sugar levels in people with type 2 diabetes. One study lasted 24 weeks, long enough to see benefits from almond consumption that included lowering of A1c, a long-term marker of blood glucose.[16]

Another study asked 34,000 Americans if they had eaten nuts in the 24 hours prior to being surveyed. Those who said yes were half as likely to have type 2 diabetes.[17]

Seeds also get into the act of helping to prevent and manage diabetes. One study found that when volunteers ate white bread that included whole or ground chia seeds, their blood sugar rose much less than when the same participants ate bread without chia. The more chia was added, the stronger the effect became.[18] And flaxseeds have also been found to aid in improving blood sugar control, even in obese patients with advanced type 2 diabetes.[19]

Nuts and Seeds May Reduce the Incidence of Gallstones

Despite their high fat content, nuts and seeds may prevent gallstones from forming. One 2004 study found that men who consumed nuts, including peanuts, had a 30 percent lower risk of developing gallstones than men who didn't eat nuts.[20]

Nuts and Seeds May Improve Sexual Health

A 2011 study gave 100 grams of pistachio nuts daily for 3 weeks to 17 men suffering from erectile dysfunction. Not only did the participants who consumed pistachios lower their total and LDL cholesterol while increasing their good HDL cholesterol, but they also significantly improved their ability to achieve and maintain erections.[21]

EASY ALMOND BUTTER RECIPE

3 cups of raw or dry roasted almonds
¼ teaspoon sea salt, optional

DIRECTIONS

Add almonds and salt to a food processor and pulse until the almonds are grainy. They should resemble a meal-like texture. Scrape down the sides of the bowl, place the lid back on the processor, and process until smooth. Depending on the brand of almonds and the strength of your food processor, this may take 3 to 8 minutes to achieve a creamy and smooth consistency.

Store in a sealed container on the counter for 2 weeks, or in the refrigerator for up to 4 weeks.

Each year, Pfizer makes more than $1.5 billion selling Viagra. The company fears competition from rival drugs like Cialis and Levitra. Perhaps it should also be a bit worried about competition from pistachio farmers!

Storing Nuts and Seeds

After buying nuts and seeds, store them in airtight containers in the refrigerator or freezer to keep their oils from going rancid. Fresh nuts are generally best. If you have a nutcracker (and some time and energy), buy walnuts in the shell and crack them as needed. You can also get them shelled, in which case you'll want to eat them right away or keep them chilled.

It's a good idea to keep your seeds refrigerated or frozen as well. You can enjoy hemp seeds right out of the package, but if you buy whole flaxseeds, you may want to grind them to to allow your body access to their nutritional bounty. I use an inexpensive coffee grinder for this job. Once I've ground a batch, I store it in the fridge in an airtight container.

Culinary Uses for Nuts and Seeds

You can enjoy nuts raw or roasted, whole or chopped or ground.

Snack on them plain, with a sprinkling of salt, or as part of a homemade trail mix.

They're delicious added to a nut loaf or casserole, blended into nut milks and smoothies, and used as the base for a "nut cheese."

You can sprinkle them over salads and stir-fries, use them in desserts (they're great when ground into a natural pie crust), or blend them into sauces, dips, and spreads. You can buy premade nut and seed butters or make your own with a food processor or high-speed blender.

NUTS AND SEEDS RECIPES

BREAKFAST

Elixir of Life Smoothie Bowl

Rockin' Rollup Lentil Sausage Breakfast Wraps

Hearty Blueberry Walnut Hotcakes

Sweet and Spice and Everything Nice Breakfast Bowl

Sweet Baked Apple Walnut Oatmeal

Warm Banana Chia Breakfast Pudding

MAINS

Plant-tastic Mushroom Ziti Bake

Mighty Greens Power Bowl

(Bring La) Fiesta Roasted Sweet Potato Bowl

Everyday Lentil Lunch

Kickin' Kimchi "Fried" Rice and Veggies

Vegged-Out Tofu Pad Thai

SALADS

Fill Me with Warmth Tempeh and Kale Salad

Uncomplicated Crunchy Kale Slaw

Lemony Basil Farro Salad

Hearty Wild Rice, Mushroom, and Baby Broccoli Salad

Minty Fresh Strawberry Salad

Feeling Upbeet and Lively Lentil Salad

Super Seed Autumn Salad with Tart Pomegranate Dressing

SOUPS/STEWS

Butter Bean Me Up One-Pot Soup

Sweet and Savory Peanut Soup

Creamy Dreamy Arugula and White Bean Soup

Sunset Glow Root Veggie Soup with Toasted Sunflower Seeds

Gourd-geous Nourishing Pumpkin Chili

SIDES

Herbaceous Wild Rice and Mushroom Stuffing

Garlicky Parmesan Broccoli

SNACKS

Enlighten Me Matcha Muffins

Zesty Chili Lime Kale Chips

Sweet and Savory Spiced Pecans

Super Seedy Granola

DESSERTS

Oh-So-Sweet Green Tea Pistachio Nice Cream

Bright and Fruity Blueberry Lemon Bars

Summertime Strawberry Rhubarb Crisp

Sweet Vitality Carrot Cake

DRINKS

Invigorating Tropical Green Smoothie

Hemp-tastic Strawberry Shortcake Smoothie

Espresso My Love of Mocha Smoothie

CHAPTER 9

COFFEE AND TEA

Once upon a time, there was an Ethiopian monk with a problem. According to legend,[1] he just couldn't stay awake during prayers, which made him look bad to his monastic brothers. One day he was traveling through a field when he happened upon a strange and wondrous sight—a pirouetting shepherd and a herd of capering goats.

Both the shepherd and his flock were dancing up a storm. Even the old buck was leaping like a little kid. The monk asked the shepherd about the fantastic dance party he was witnessing and soon discovered that both man and goats had been feasting on the berries of a nearby coffee bush.

The monk, realizing that he had found the solution to his sleepiness, picked handfuls of berries, stuffed his pockets, and continued on his journey. When he returned to the monastery, he reconstituted the now-dried berries by boiling them and drinking the liquid.

As a result, this particular monk became a model of energetic piety, and it wasn't long before the other monks were also using the wondrous bean to power their own spiritual quests.

Separated from the Ethiopian monk by many miles and many centuries, the Chinese emperor Shen Nung was traveling with his entourage when he decided to camp under a tea tree. The heat from a cooking fire dried some leaves, which fell into a pot of boiling water and produced a heavenly scent. Upon drinking the water, the emperor was struck by the delicious taste and the invigorating effect on his body. And so was discovered tea.[2]

And those, I'd like to think, are the origin stories of two of the world's most popular beverages.

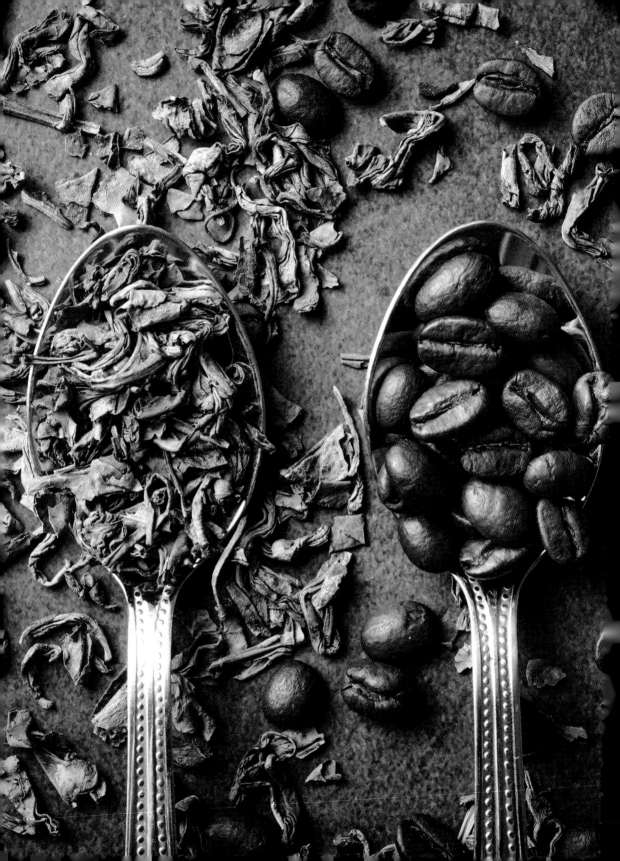

Unlike some of the superfoods in this book, coffee and tea don't need a marketing agency to get people to consume them. Billions of people around the world fuel their lives with coffee, and tea is the second most popular drink in the world in gallons drunk per day, topped only by water.

Despite their popularity, coffee and tea often get a bad rap among the health conscious. Sure, they make you feel good when you drink them. Sure, they give you energy and focus (at least the caffeinated varieties). But in a culture that teaches us that whatever feels good must be bad for you (I'm looking at you, donuts), all pleasures are seen as guilty ones.

So I'm happy to report that the preponderance of scientific data is fairly clear: both coffee and tea, consumed in moderation, can be health-promoting superfoods for most people.

It's taken me many years to accept the evidence. I didn't grow up drinking coffee or caffeinated tea, and for a long time, I thought that my dad's single cup of coffee every morning was his own guilty pleasure—a singular indulgence enjoyed by a man of self-discipline and resolve. That said, I've always loved the conversations we have after he's consumed his morning joe. I know I'm biased, but this brilliant and amazing man is even more brilliant and amazing when fueled by a high-quality brew.

Now I see that cuppa as an integral part of his health regimen, stimulating both the cognitive and mood centers of the brain. In his mid-70s, my dad is as sharp and loving as ever, and science says that coffee may help him stay that way for many more years.

I, too, appreciate the pleasures of coffee, although I rarely partake, because I find that even though I enjoy the initial sensations, I tend to get jittery and even irritable a few hours later. So although there are a lot of reasons to drink coffee, there are definitely people—like me—for whom it's not a great idea. If your body doesn't do well with coffee, you can get most if not all the benefits from decaffeinated varieties, or from other foods and beverages.

Tea—and I should say "teas," because there are huge differences between black, green, and white teas; matcha; and herbal varieties—is also a health booster and mood lifter. There are teas with caffeine, which all come from *Camellia sinensis*, the tea plant. And there are teas made from the leaves and flowers of other plants, including chamomile, hibiscus, lavender, and mint. Each plant offers its own set of health-promoting properties.

Coffee provides fuel for activity, ambition, and drive, and so is best suited as a morning beverage. Health experts typically advise avoiding coffee after 3:00 pm (for those working day shifts), because the caffeine can remain in your system for hours and interfere with your sleep.

Tea, on the other hand, can be a wonderful afternoon and evening beverage. Whether the British afternoon tea (enjoyed by upper classes as they relaxed in comfortable parlor chairs) or high tea (taken by workers done with their labors), or in the elaborately mindful Japanese tea ceremonies, people have traditionally used tea to slow down, savor life, and simply enjoy what they already have.

Both types of beverages can support our physical, mental, and emotional health, in different ways and at different times of day. Coffee reminds us that we are creatures of action, able to change the world. Tea allows us to pause, reflect, and appreciate the world as it is.

What Are Coffee and Tea?

Coffee is a drink made from roasted coffee beans, which are actually the seeds of berries from a variety of *Coffea* plant, which is native to tropical regions of Asia and Africa. There are two main varieties of *Coffea* plant: arabica and robusta.[3] Arabica coffee is considered to be higher quality than robusta. Unfortunately, the plants are more delicate and harder to grow, and therefore more labor-intensive and expensive. Robusta is higher in caffeine, which acts as a natural pest repellent. Robusta coffee beans typically end up in cheap coffee, including many discount instant varieties, where its "robust" (some say "harsh") taste can be masked by the addition of lots of sugar and cream.

The tea plant is an evergreen shrub native to East Asia. Many varieties of tea come from this one plant; the leaves and leaf buds can be turned into black, green, white, yellow, matcha, and green teas, as well as pu-erh and oolong varieties. They vary in how long the leaves are left on the plant before harvesting, as well as how they are processed.

Processing generally involves allowing the leaves to oxidize, either partially (in the case of oolong) or fully (as is done for black tea), and applying various kinds of heat in different intensities at different times in the process. Herbal teas are those made from plants other than the tea plant. Popular herbal teas include those made from flowers (chamomile, rose, jasmine, and lavender), leaves (mint, passionflower, lemon balm, and rooibos), and roots (ginger and dandelion).

On the island where I grew up, you could find and harvest wild herbs to make calming, nutrient-rich, and delicious teas. Chamomile, mint, and nettle teas were staples of my childhood.

Coffee and Tea Nutrition

The best-known nutrient in coffee (and nonherbal tea) is caffeine, which acts as a stimulant on your central nervous system. It's also been shown to reduce inflammation, a condition at the root of most chronic diseases.

Both coffee and tea are rich in anti-oxidants such as catechins, polyphenols, vitamin C, and tannins. Green tea in particular is a potent source of a catechin with the heroic-sounding name of epigallocatechin gallate (EGCG), which can prevent the formation of free radicals in your cells. Matcha tea, which is powdered so you consume all of the leaf rather than just getting the nutrients that dissolve into hot water, has about three times the antioxidants of regular green tea.

Adding lemon to your tea can boost antioxidant availability, while dairy can decrease it.

Why Coffee and Tea Deserve Superfood Status

Before I share research on the health benefits of coffee and tea, I want to put that research in context. Many of the remarkable benefits of coffee and tea appear to be due to the large variety and amounts of antioxidants those beverages contain. The problem is, most people eating a modern industrialized diet aren't getting many antioxidants from other sources. In fact, it's estimated that the average American gets fully half of their antioxidants from coffee alone.

So we know that people who are practically starved for antioxidants benefit immensely from coffee and tea. What we don't know is how great the benefit is for those already consuming abundant antioxidants from a varied, minimally processed, plant-based diet.

A second bit of important context is that many people take their coffee and tea full of ingredients that aren't great for their health: sugar, artificial sweeteners, milk, cream, and artificial creamers. So it's possible that coffee and tea are even better for your health than the studies suggest.

And thirdly, it's important to state, again, that not everyone does well with caffeine. Some people find that it makes them jittery, anxious, and stressed out. And many find that it negatively impacts their sleep. So as in all things, but especially so with caffeinated beverages—listen to your body and do what makes sense and feels best to you.

Now with those caveats in place, let's look at what the studies tell us.

Coffee and Tea Support Cardiovascular Health

Because coffee causes your blood vessels to expand, it's good for your circulation.[4] And that means your heart doesn't have to pump as hard, and plaques are less likely to turn into stroke-causing blood clots. A 2009 study of 83,000 female American nurses reported that coffee drinking may "modestly reduce" the risk of stroke in women.[5] A 2011 study of 34,000 Swedish women replicated and strengthened this result, finding that those who drank less than one cup of coffee per day had an increased risk of stroke.[6] And a 2018 article estimated that drinking 3 to 5 cups per day could lower your risk of cardiovascular disease by 15 percent.[7]

Caffeinated tea also appears to support a healthy heart and circulatory system.[8] A 2009 study published in the *Journal of Hypertension* (can you imagine how stressed-out those editors must get as their deadline approaches?) found that black tea given to healthy men improved a metric called flow-mediated dilation.[9] This just means that black tea helps arteries expand to accommodate greater blood flow, which is a good thing if you want to avoid high blood pressure.

Green tea is also a potent heart helper. Its polyphenols support a healthy endothelium, the all-important lining of your blood vessels. While endothelial function typically degrades as you age, drinking copious amounts of green tea can dramatically slow the decline. Not only that, green tea can help lower total and "bad" LDL cholesterol.[10] A Japanese study that followed 40,000 healthy men for 11 years found that those who drank green tea had a significantly reduced risk of dying from cardiovascular disease.[11]

Teas Can Help You Rest and Relax

Just as coffee tends to pump you up, tea can help you downshift. Several popular herbal teas—chamomile, lavender, lemon balm, and valerian, among others—have been linked to better sleep.[12]

And you might be surprised to learn that matcha, which contains caffeine, also can help you relax. That's thanks to its high levels of L-theanine, an amino acid that can support a calm and meditative state that's perfect for deep focus.[13]

Coffee and Tea Can Support Your Immune System

All those antioxidants in coffee and tea may help your body fight off infection, and even prevent sun damage to skin. Coffee contains a polyphenol called chlorogenic acid that can neutralize free radicals and keep them from damaging your cells. It also protects the immune system against attack from a class of compounds called reactive oxygen species.[14]

Tea is also no slouch when it comes to immune support. Your body can convert that peaceful amino acid L-theanine into ethylamine, which can prime some of the T cells of your immune system to react faster and more aggressively to potential diseases and infections.[15]

Coffee and Tea May Prevent Cancer

Green tea, rich in EGCG and other catechins, has long been studied for its anticancer properties. A 2018 paper shared data suggesting that one of the mechanisms by which green tea can help prevent cancer is by disrupting the ability of cancer stem cells to divide and turn into other kinds of cells.[16]

Caffeine may also reduce cancer risk by suppressing inflammation, which is a driver of some cancers.[17] The American Cancer Society reports that coffee may decrease the incidence of head and neck, colorectal, breast, and liver cancers.[18]

Coffee and Tea Decrease Risk of Dementia and Parkinson's Disease

One of the most-studied effects of coffee and other caffeinated beverages is their ability to keep your brain healthy as you age. As a vasodilator, caffeine can increase blood flow to your brain, stimulating it to be more active in the short term and protecting it from damage in the long term.

This is more than just theory. The Cardiovascular Risk Factors, Aging and Dementia study out of Finland, which tracked more than 1,400 people for over two decades, found that those who drank 3 to 5 cups of coffee per day at midlife had a reduced risk of developing dementia by a whopping 65 percent.[19]

In addition to dementia, coffee and tea appear protective against another neuro-degenerative disease, Parkinson's. A 2007 study reported that drinking 5 or more cups of coffee per day was associated with a 60 percent reduction in Parkinson's Disease.[20] Three or more cups of tea achieved the same result. The researchers didn't say what would happen if someone drank both coffee *and* tea in those quantities every day;

presumably, they'd be too busy running to the toilet to complete the questionnaire.

Green tea in particular has been shown to help reduce the risk of neurodegenerative diseases such as Alzheimer's and Parkinson's. Medical journals often end their discussions of the benefits by suggesting that the compounds in green tea "could be useful for the development of new drugs."[21] My take is, why wait? Take advantage of its goodness and drink green tea now.

Caffeine Can Help You Be More Active

If exercise were a pill, it would be considered one of the great blockbuster drugs of all time. It's one of the most studied and most effective health interventions ever. And unlike medication, the side effects of physical activity can be wholly positive (as long as you move responsibly and don't hurt yourself). Exercise can help reduce the risk of cardiovascular disease, stroke, cancer, type 2 diabetes, and osteoporosis. It improves brain function and mental health. And it enhances mood and energy levels.

Unfortunately for the drug companies (but fortunately for you!), exercise isn't a pill or anything for which to bill insurance companies—in fact it doesn't have to cost a dime. And a piece of good news for people who know they "should" exercise but feel too fatigued to do so is that caffeine can help them be more active. A 2018 Australian study looked at coffee and tea intake in a group of 7,500 middle-aged women and correlated it with their levels of physical activity.[22] Those women who reported drinking 1 to 2 cups of coffee or tea per day were more likely to be physically active than those who drank less. Interestingly, only the coffee drinkers reported feeling less tired and more energetic; the tea drinkers, while still exercising more, didn't have the same subjective experience of increased energy. (I'm thinking the placebo effect may have been at play here; we tend to think of coffee and not tea as a pick-me-up).

Buying and Storing Coffee and Tea

You can buy coffee in dozens of different ways. There's instant, dry ground, roasted and unroasted whole beans, canned, bottled, and steaming cups to go from your local coffee shop. There are machines that allow you to buy their cartridges, add water, flip a switch, and have everything done for you. You can also become your own barista, using a pour-over style glass coffee maker like a Chemex or far more elaborate and expensive pieces of equipment. If you're really into coffee and have a fair amount of disposable income, you can get your very own espresso machine for anywhere from a few hundred to tens of thousands of dollars.

The cold brew method, in which you steep coffee for up to 24 hours in cold or room temperature water and then strain, is a great way to reduce the bitterness and acidity in coffee.[23]

Store whole coffee beans in an airtight container away from moisture, heat, and light. Roasted beans begin losing flavor and freshness right away, so buy them in small batches and try to use them up within a few weeks. Ground coffee degrades even faster because the grounds' increased surface area exposes them to more oxygen. You can freeze coffee beans and grounds in an airtight container to keep them fresh longer.

There are two main ways to purchase tea: dried and bottled. You can get dried tea both bagged and loose-leaf. If you're really into the ritual of brewing tea, loose-leaf varieties will allow you to participate more in the process: measuring the leaves and placing them in a brew basket or strainer to steep. Some specialty teas come only in loose-leaf form. For most people, tea bags are fine and require less effort, time, and commitment to the process.

Store tea in an airtight container in a dark, cool, dry place.[24] Oxygen is the enemy of tea leaf longevity, unless the leaves were fully oxidized during the manufacturing process. Oolong and black teas will degrade more slowly than the less oxidized green and white varieties. Heat and light also degrade leaves faster. Avoid humidity, as that will cause the leaves to steep a bit, releasing their flavor into the moist air as if they were already steeping in water. And don't store tea next to strong odors as the leaves can absorb those scents (unless you're excited about garlic oolong).

PROS AND CONS OF TANNINS

Tannins are a class of chemicals found in plants. Specifically, they're part of the family of polyphenols, many of which are celebrated for their amazing health benefits.

PROS	CONS
Antioxidant Capabilities: Help to reduce oxidative damage	Potentially block the absorption of nutrients: If you consume your coffee or tea with a serving of vitamin C-rich fruit you mitigate these effects. Consider drinking tea between meals rather than with meals to avoid it blocking nutrient absorption.
Balance Blood Pressure and Lower Cholesterol	Tannin Sensitivity: Apply heat to reduce concentrations and steep your tea for shorter periods of time.
Antiviral and Antimicrobial Activity	
Anti-inflammatory	

Bottled tea is often little more than sugar water. Lipton's Lemon Iced Tea, for example, contains 32 grams of added sugar per 2.5 cup serving.[25] If you drink bottled teas, look for varieties with little or no added sugar.

Culinary Uses for Coffee and Tea

There are healthy and unhealthy ways to take your coffee and tea. One way to make tea and coffee far less healthy is to add lots of sugar and cream. Remember that both are acquired tastes for most people, so you can retrain your taste buds to appreciate unsweetened or lightly sweetened coffee or tea.

And if you really enjoy the creaminess that comes from milk, cream, or nondairy creamer, try using a plant milk. There are dozens of different varieties and brands available now, from soy to oat to hemp to cashew to almond to coconut. But these can get expensive and also produce a lot of packaging waste, so if you're committed to plant milk, you might want to start making your own. A blender and strainer cloth is all you need, although you can automate the process with a dedicated plant milk maker like an Almond Cow or ChefWave. For tea, try it plain, with a squeeze of lemon, or flavored with sliced ginger or another herbal tea. If you find that unpalatable, add just a dab of your favorite sweetener and see if you can slowly reduce the amount over time. I love my matcha with a bit of unsweetened soy milk. It reminds me that not everything in life is supposed to be sweet, and that I can enjoy—and not merely endure—the bitter.

For the sweet spot in terms of health benefits, try to drink 1 to 4 cups a day; experiment to find the amount and types that work best for you.

In addition to drinking coffee and tea on their own, you can also use them in a variety of beverage recipes, desserts, and even sauces.

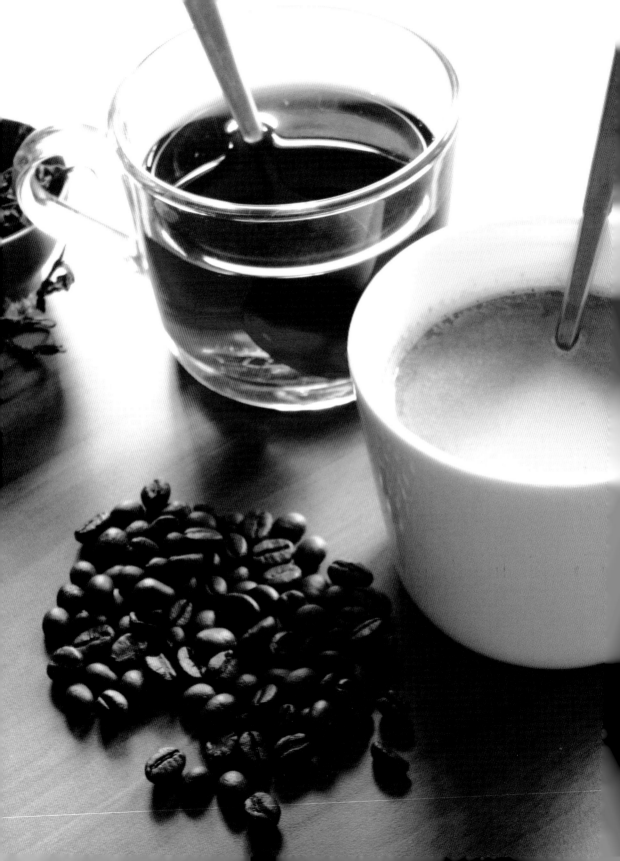

COFFEE & TEA RECIPES

SNACKS

Enlighten Me Matcha Muffins

DESSERTS

Oh-So-Sweet Green Tea Pistachio Nice Cream

DRINKS

Cool as a Cucumber Matcha Refresher
Enchanting Masala Chai
Mindfulness Moment Matcha Tea
Espresso My Love of Mocha Smoothie

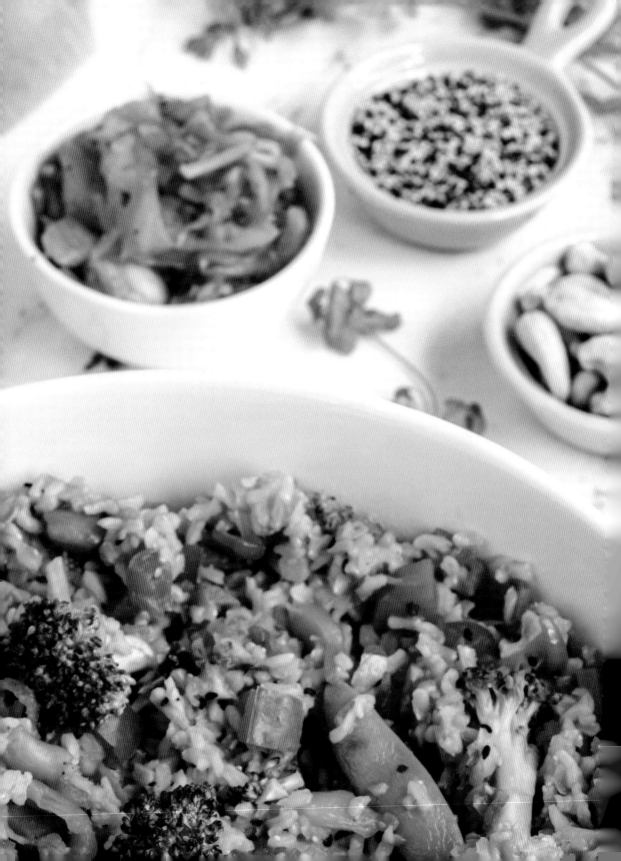

PART TWO

REAL SUPERFOODS RECIPES

SUPERFOOD GROUPS

AT A GLANCE

 LEAFY GREENS

 MUSHROOMS

 LEGUMES

 BERRIES

 ALLIUMS

 HERBS AND SPICES

 SWEET POTATOES

 NUTS AND SEEDS

 COFFEE AND TEA

Now that you're a Real Superfoods Expert, it's time to roll up your sleeves in the kitchen. The recipes that follow will make it super easy to get these superfoods into yourself and your loved ones. They're delicious (that's what our taste testers have told us!), and each highlights at least one, and usually multiple, Real Superfoods.

While one goal of this book is to boost your superfood consumption, another is to keep unhealthy ingredients out of your diet. That's why all of the recipes in this book are 100 percent plant-based. They don't use processed sugar, relying instead on whole food sweeteners like dates and bananas (and occasionally maple syrup). You can also make all the recipes without added oil or salt—even in recipes where they appear in small amounts, those ingredients are totally optional. If you're avoiding gluten, we've got you covered as well, with gluten-free substitutions in every case.

A Few Culinary Notes

A bunch of recipes call for smoked paprika; it's not the same as sweet or Hungarian hot varieties. To get the most flavor in these dishes, it's worth your while to find the genuine smoked spice.

You'll also see something called "nutritional yeast" in some savory recipes. If you're not familiar with the yellow flakes, you might think something with that name must taste as grim as it sounds. So you'll be delighted to discover that "nooch," as many

chefs affectionately call it, is kind of cheesy, full of umami, and equally delightful as a condiment, spice, and topping.

While we don't explicitly call for organic ingredients, you may want to choose organic if you can find it and they fit your budget. There's increasing evidence that organic produce is healthier than conventional for the consumer, and definitely so for the farm worker who's exposed to whatever is being applied to their crops.

We also recommend that in the recipes that call for canned foods (typically tomatoes), you choose BPA-free cans whenever possible. BPA is an endocrine-disrupting chemical that is known for leaching from can liners into food, so choosing cans (or cartons) that don't contain the chemical will help protect you from its toxic effects.

Several recipes include plant milk. There are many different types these days: soy, oat, almond, flax, hemp, rice, and cashew. They vary in taste, consistency, and price, so go with whatever works best for you. Just check the label to make sure whatever version you get is unsweetened.

One last thing before we get cooking: you'll see icons identifying each of the superfood groups alongside each recipe, so you can tell at a glance which superfoods are in it. The icons are shown on page 122, so you can get familiar with them before diving in.

Okay, that's enough talk. It's time to get cooking!

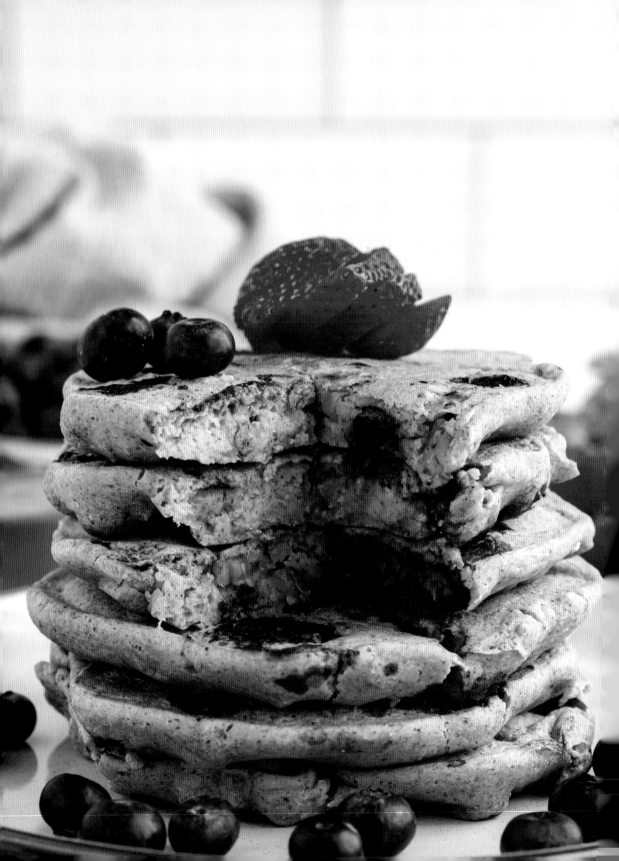

BALANCED
BREAKFAST DISHES

ELIXIR OF LIFE SMOOTHIE BOWL

Set yourself up for an energized, plant-strong day with organic spinach, protein-rich hemp seeds, creamy banana, and fudgy dates blended in perfect harmony. The result is a delightful green smoothie bowl that will put a smile on your face and health in your heart. Top with rolled oats, sesame seeds, and even cacao nibs for a chocolatey experience.

Serves 2 **Prep time** 10 minutes **Cooking time** none

Smoothie Bowl Base

2 fresh or frozen ripe bananas
¼ cup hulled hemp seeds
¼ cup unsweetened plant-based milk, or more if needed
¼ cup tahini
4 pitted dates
2 handfuls spinach
1 teaspoon ground cinnamon
2 pinches salt, optional

Toppings

2 tablespoons unsweetened cacao nibs, optional
2 tablespoons sesame seeds
¼ cup raw rolled oats

1. Blend the smoothie base ingredients until mostly smooth. You may have some small pieces of dates in there, which can make it delicious; but if you want it really smooth, keep blending. Add 1 to 2 tablespoons of plant-based milk until the desired consistency is reached.
2. Divide the mixture between two bowls.
3. Sprinkle the cacao nibs, sesame seeds, and rolled oats on top.

CHEF'S NOTES

Substitutions

Use chia seeds in place of hemp seeds (you might need more liquid, as the chia will absorb quite a bit).

Use almond butter, peanut butter, or cashew butter in place of tahini.

Substitute another leafy green of choice in place of spinach, like romaine or kale.

Instead of cacao nibs, use unsweetened shredded coconut.

Substitute sunflower, pumpkin seeds, or chia seeds in place of sesame seeds.

Storage

Prepare the base ahead of time and store it in an airtight container in the refrigerator for up to 3 days. Note that you may have to re-blend the smoothie and add more milk or water to reach the desired consistency.

Store the leftover base, without the toppings, in an airtight container in the refrigerator for up to 3 days.

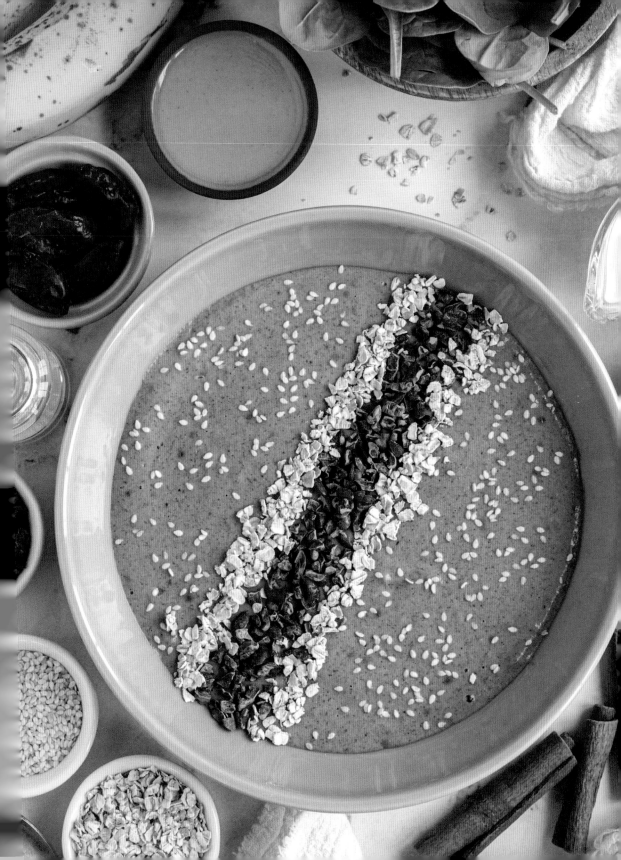

ROCKIN' ROLLUP LENTIL SAUSAGE BREAKFAST WRAPS

If savory breakfast foods are your jam and fragrant spices are your dream, then these quick-cooking wraps may become your new breakfast staple. We do recommend the hot sauce for moisture and spice. If spiciness isn't your thing, then try a mild salsa or pico de gallo, or a creamy plant-based sauce like the Cauliflower Squash Cheese Sauce (page 160).

Serves 2 **Prep time** 15 minutes **Cooking time** 5 minutes

Lentil Sausage

½ cup walnuts, optional

2 cups cooked brown or green lentils

2 teaspoons fresh sage, roughly minced

1 teaspoon onion powder

½ teaspoon garlic powder

1 teaspoon dried oregano

2 teaspoons smoked or regular paprika

¼ teaspoon salt, optional

¼ teaspoon black pepper, optional

2 tablespoons fresh parsley, minced

Wrap

4 collard green leaves

½ cup tomatoes, diced

¼ cup red onion, diced

¼ cup fresh cilantro, roughly minced (optional)

Hot sauce or other condiment of your choice

1. Toast the walnuts, if using. Add the walnuts to a large skillet and heat on medium for 2 minutes, tossing occasionally to prevent them from burning.
2. Add the lentils, sage, onion powder, garlic powder, oregano, paprika, and optional salt and pepper to the skillet. Stir until well combined.
3. Add ¼ cup of water and parsley, stir, and continue to cook the sausage ingredients until the water is absorbed, about 1 minute.
4. Remove the mixture from the heat and transfer it to a food processor. Pulse 4 to 5 times until the lentils and walnuts are just about, but not quite, pureed.
5. Lay out your collard leaves and divide the lentil "sausage" between the four wraps, forming a line with the lentils down the middle of the wrap.
6. Divide the tomatoes, onions, and optional cilantro between the four leaves.
7. Add a little hot sauce, if desired, or your favorite plant-based sauce or salsa over the top of each.
8. Fold each short end of the wrap inward about 1 inch toward the center. Then, starting with one long edge of the greens, tightly roll the wraps around the contents to form a (rockin') rollup.

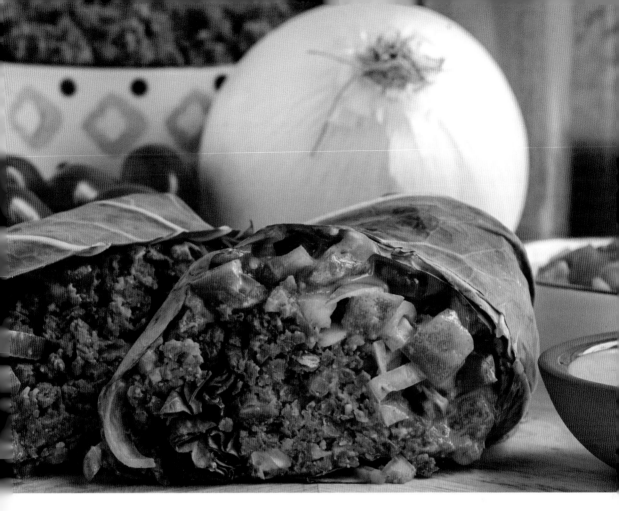

CHEF'S NOTES

Substitutions

Substitute a legume of choice for the lentils, such as kidney beans or black beans.

Use red bell peppers in place of tomatoes.

Instead of collard greens, use organic Swiss chard, romaine, or kale.

Use another herb like parsley, basil, or chives in place of cilantro.

Make It Spicy

Add 1 or 2 dashes of cayenne pepper or red pepper flakes to the mixture before blending it in the food processor.

Keep It Nut Free

Omit the walnuts and either substitute ½ cup of sunflower seeds for the walnuts or add an additional ½ cup of lentils.

Storage

Store leftover lentil sausage in an airtight container in the refrigerator for up to 5 days or freeze it for up to one month.

HEARTY BLUEBERRY WALNUT HOTCAKES

Blueberries provide natural sweetness and walnuts deliver crunchy texture and nutty flavor to these pancakes, which will keep you full throughout the morning thanks to the healthy omega-3 fats in the flax meal, protein in the hemp seeds, and fiber in the oats. Since flax meal absorbs liquid (and can turn into a rock if it sits too long), it's best to make the pancakes immediately after mixing the batter rather than keeping extra batter in the refrigerator.

Serves 2 **Prep time** 10 minutes **Cooking time** 10 minutes

1 medium banana

1 cup rolled oats

½ cup unsweetened plant-based milk

1 tablespoon hemp seeds

1 tablespoon ground flax meal

1 tablespoon maple syrup

1 teaspoon baking powder

1 tablespoon apple cider vinegar

1 teaspoon vanilla extract

Pinch of salt, optional

½ cup blueberries

¼ cup walnuts, chopped

1. Add all the ingredients, except the blueberries and walnuts, to a food processor or blender and blend for 2 to 3 minutes until smooth.

2. Transfer the mixture to a medium bowl and stir in the blueberries and walnuts.

3. Spoon the pancake mixture onto a griddle, over medium heat, to form 4-inch-round pancakes, which will give you approximately 8 pancakes total. Depending on your griddle, you may need a bit of vegetable oil to prevent the pancakes from sticking.

4. Cook on each side until the bottom is golden brown and bubbles break the surface of the pancakes.

5. Top the pancakes with more nutritional goodness, if you'd like. See Chef's Notes for ideas!

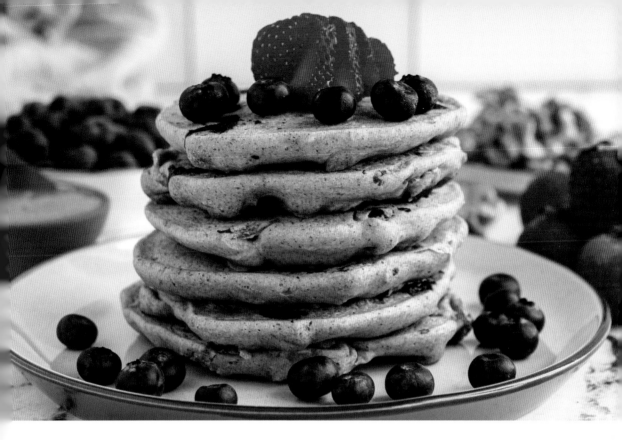

CHEF'S NOTES

Substitutions

Use organic apples, organic peaches, or a different organic berry in place of the blueberries.

Use pecan or almond pieces in place of walnuts.

Keep It Simple

If you don't have blueberries or walnuts, this recipe is delicious without them. But they do add more nutritional value!

Layer It Up

Add fresh fruit on top.

Top with your favorite nut or seed butter.

Add cinnamon or nutmeg to the batter for a little spicy deliciousness.

Storage

Flax meal absorbs liquid, so any leftover batter will get pretty thick if it's stored overnight. It's best to cook any remaining batter and store the hotcake leftovers in an airtight container in the refrigerator (for up to 5 days) or in the freezer (for up to one month). If you do store batter overnight in the fridge, simply add more milk until you get the desired consistency again before cooking.

EASY PEASY TOFU BREAKFAST BITES

These little muffin bites are light, airy, and bursting with flavor from mushrooms, spices, and herbs. Also, it's a lot of fun to eat tofu as a muffin! These keep well in the refrigerator and reheat quickly in a toaster oven or regular oven for a quick and sustaining breakfast or snack throughout the day.

Serves 6 to 8 **Prep time** 10 minutes **Cooking time** 35 minutes

Sautéed Vegetables

1 cup red, white, or yellow onion, chopped

2 cups button, cremini, or portobello mushrooms, chopped

1 teaspoon ground turmeric

1 teaspoon onion powder

1 teaspoon oregano

¼ teaspoon salt, optional

¼ teaspoon black pepper, optional

2 cups kale, stems removed and chopped

2 tablespoons fresh basil, finely chopped (optional)

Tofu

14 ounces firm or extra firm organic tofu, drained

¼ cup unsweetened plant-based milk

3 tablespoons nutritional yeast

1 tablespoon reduced-sodium tamari or coconut aminos

¾ teaspoon mustard powder

¼ teaspoon salt, optional

¼ teaspoon black pepper, optional

1. Preheat the oven to 375°F. Line mini muffin tins with paper liners.

2. Heat a large pan over medium-high heat. Add the onions, stirring frequently, and cook them until they are translucent, about 2 to 3 minutes.

3. Add 2 to 4 tablespoons of water to deglaze the pan, turn the heat down to medium, stir in the mushrooms, and cook for another 2 to 3 minutes, stirring occasionally.

4. Add the turmeric, onion powder, oregano, and optional salt and black pepper. Mix well so the spices coat the vegetables.

5. Stir in the kale and optional basil until the kale is slightly wilted (about 30 to 60 seconds). Turn off the heat and set aside.

6. In a food processor, add the tofu, milk, nutritional yeast, tamari, mustard powder, and optional salt and pepper. Blend until smooth.

7. Pour the tofu mixture into the vegetable mixture and stir until the tofu and vegetables are combined.

8. Fill each muffin cup to the top with the tofu-vegetable mixture. This recipe should make approximately 24 mini muffins.

9. Bake the muffins for 30 to 35 minutes, until they are golden brown on top. Let them sit for 10 minutes before serving.

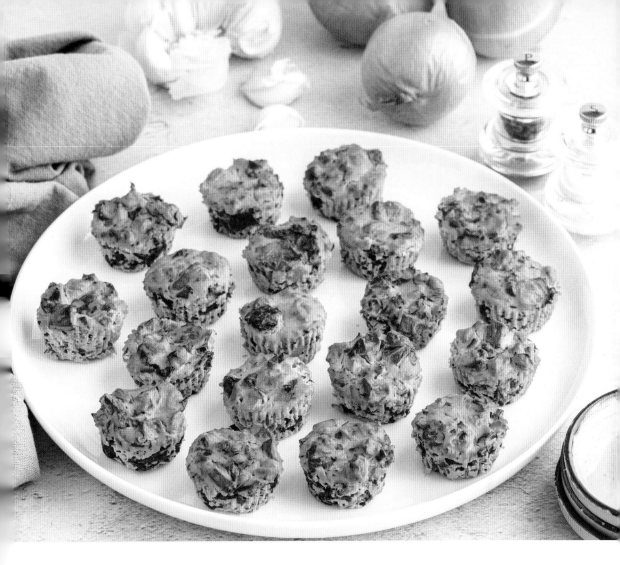

CHEF'S NOTES

Substitutions

Use other vegetables of your choice, such as broccoli, red bell pepper, or spinach in place of the mushrooms and kale.

Use chopped shallots in place of the chopped onion.

Use onion granules in place of onion powder.

Prep Ahead

Make the tofu mixture ahead of time and store it in the fridge for up to 24 hours before using.

Storage

Store leftovers in an airtight container in the refrigerator for up to 5 days.

NO MUSS, NO FUSS BREAKFAST BURRITO

One-sheet meals are all the rage for good reason—they're simple to prepare and require little cleanup, making them efficient and (typically) stress-free breakfast options. If you're a fan of hearty morning meals, then this breakfast burrito has you covered. It's packed with protein from the tofu and beans; fiber from the whole grain tortilla, avocado, and beans; and phytonutrients from the herbs, spices, leafy greens and . . . beans! This is one nutritionally complete breakfast to help you power through your morning.

Serves 2 **Prep time** 15 minutes **Cooking time** 25 minutes

Sheet Pan Ingredients

8 ounces firm or extra firm organic tofu, drained

1½ teaspoons ground turmeric

½ teaspoon onion powder

½ teaspoon smoked paprika

¼ teaspoon salt, optional

¼ teaspoon black pepper, optional

½ large red bell pepper, stemmed, seeded, and thinly sliced

½ small red onion, cut into thin strips

Burrito

2 burrito-sized whole grain tortillas or gluten-free tortillas of choice

1 cup organic spinach, chopped

1 cup home-cooked or canned black beans, rinsed and drained

½ large avocado, sliced into strips

Organic salsa or hot sauce of your choice

¼ cup fresh cilantro, roughly minced (optional)

1. Preheat the oven to 375°F and line a baking sheet with parchment paper.
2. Crumble the tofu into a medium bowl. Add the turmeric, onion powder, smoked paprika, and optional salt and pepper. Stir well until the tofu is coated in the spice mixture.
3. On one half of the baking sheet, evenly spread out the tofu mixture.
4. On the other half of the baking sheet, evenly spread out the peppers and onions. Sprinkle them with a little salt and pepper, if desired.
5. Bake for 25 minutes, tossing both the tofu and vegetables halfway through.
6. Once the tofu and vegetables are done baking, warm the tortillas on a griddle on low-medium heat. Heat on each side for about 1 to 2 minutes before transferring the tortillas to two separate plates.
7. Divide the spinach between the two tortillas, then layer the tofu, peppers and onions, beans, avocado, salsa or hot sauce, and optional cilantro in the center of each tortilla.
8. To make a burrito, first fold the bottom of the tortilla toward the center. Then fold the top down toward the center. Fold one side into the center and roll to make a burrito!

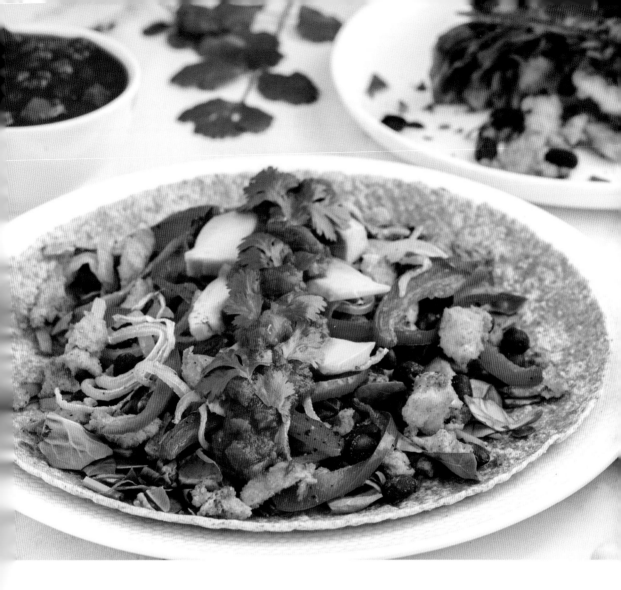

CHEF'S NOTES

Substitutions

Instead of spinach, use another leafy green of your choice.

In place of red bell pepper, use yellow, green, or orange bell peppers.

Instead of red onion, use yellow or white onion.

Substitute collard or romaine greens for your wraps instead of tortillas.

Storage

Store leftover filling in an airtight container in the refrigerator for up to 3 days.

SWEET AND SPICE AND EVERYTHING NICE BREAKFAST BOWL

This wouldn't be a superfood cookbook without sweet potatoes. These naturally sweet orange jewels are power-packed with carotenes and fiber. We like banana, cinnamon, pecans, and almond butter as toppings, but this is where you can let your creativity shine and choose any that sound scrumptious to you (oats, pumpkin seeds, and dates come to mind). This bowl feels extra comforting on a crisp autumn day!

Serves 2 **Prep time** 10 minutes **Cooking time** 60 minutes

Sweet Potato Base

2 medium sweet potatoes
½ cup unsweetened plant-based milk
2 tablespoons ground flax meal
2 teaspoons vanilla extract
1 teaspoon ground cinnamon
2 pinches ground nutmeg
Pinch of salt, optional

Toppings

1 large banana, sliced
½ teaspoon ground cinnamon
1 teaspoon maple syrup
2 to 4 tablespoons chopped pecans
2 tablespoons almond butter or nut butter of choice

1. Preheat the oven to 400°F. Pierce the sweet potatoes 3 to 4 times with a fork and place them on a parchment-lined baking sheet.
2. Bake for 45 to 60 minutes or until they're tender (total time will depend on the size of the potatoes). Alternatively, you could boil or microwave them, but they won't be as naturally sweet.
3. Once the potatoes are tender, remove them from the oven and allow them to cool before removing the skin.
4. Add 2 cups of the sweet potatoes to a blender or food processor, along with the milk, flax, vanilla, cinnamon, nutmeg, and optional salt. Blend until smooth. Set aside.
5. Heat a medium pan on medium-high. Add the sliced banana, and cook it while stirring frequently for 30 to 60 seconds.
6. Add the cinnamon and maple syrup to the pan. Stir well so that the bananas are completely coated. Reduce the heat to low-medium, and cook the bananas for another 3 to 4 minutes, stirring occasionally.
7. Divide the creamy sweet potato mixture between two bowls. Top with the bananas, as well as the pecans and almond butter. Stir and enjoy!

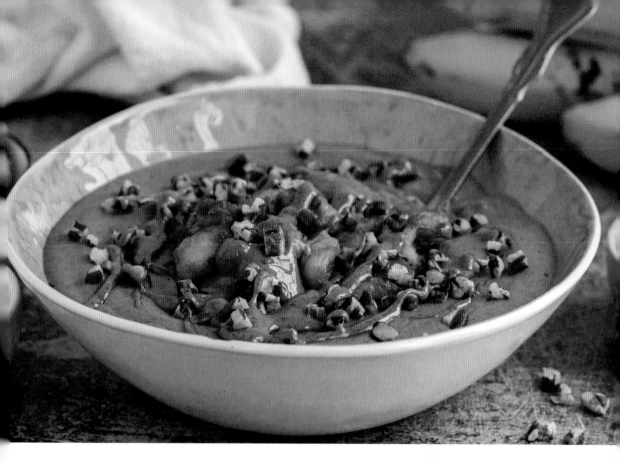

CHEF'S NOTES

Substitutions

Instead of sweet potato, use pumpkin or butternut squash.

In place of almond butter, use peanut butter, cashew butter, or sunflower butter.

Substitute another nut of choice like walnuts, almonds, or pistachios in place of pecans.

Add More Deliciousness

Sprinkle unsweetened shredded coconut on top.

Add hemp or chia seeds.

Toss in blueberries or chopped figs.

Keep It Nut Free

Use pumpkin seeds or sunflower seeds in place of pecans.

Use sunflower butter in place of almond butter.

Prep Ahead

Bake the sweet potatoes ahead of time and store them in the refrigerator for up to 3 days.

Storage

Store the sweet potato base in an airtight container in the refrigerator for up to 3 days. We recommend not adding the toppings until you're ready to eat.

SWEET BAKED APPLE WALNUT OATMEAL

This dish has a unique texture—somewhere between oatmeal and a cake! It's a little gooey (in the best way) inside hot out of the oven. If you let it sit for 10 to 15 minutes after baking, it will cook through a bit more. So plan accordingly depending on whether you like it ooey-gooey or more fully baked!

Serves 4 **Prep time** 10 minutes **Cooking time** 30 minutes

Chia Egg Substitute

2 tablespoons chia seeds
6 tablespoons water

Wet Ingredients

1 cup unsweetened plant-based milk
2 tablespoons apple cider vinegar
½ cup ripe banana, mashed
½ cup unsweetened applesauce
2 teaspoons vanilla extract

Dry Ingredients

2 cups rolled oats
¼ cup almond meal
¼ cup coconut sugar
2 teaspoons baking powder
2 teaspoons ground cinnamon
¼ teaspoon ground ginger
¼ teaspoon ground nutmeg
2 pinches salt, optional
1 cup organic apples, chopped
1 cup walnuts, chopped

1. Preheat the oven to 350°F. Line four 4-inch ramekins with pieces of parchment paper or lightly spray or coat them with oil. Alternatively, you could use silicone muffin pans or muffin pans with paper liners.
2. Add the chia seeds and 6 tablespoons of water to a small bowl, stir, and set aside. This mixture acts as a binder in place of eggs.
3. In a medium bowl, mix together the milk, apple cider vinegar, banana, applesauce, and vanilla.
4. In a large bowl, mix together the rolled oats, almond meal, coconut sugar, baking powder, cinnamon, ginger, nutmeg, and optional salt.
5. Combine the wet ingredients with the dry ingredients. Mix until combined, but don't overmix.
6. Fold in the chia egg followed by the apples and walnuts.
7. Evenly divide the batter into the ramekins and bake for 30 minutes (or 25 minutes if using muffin pans).
8. Allow to cool for 5 minutes before serving.

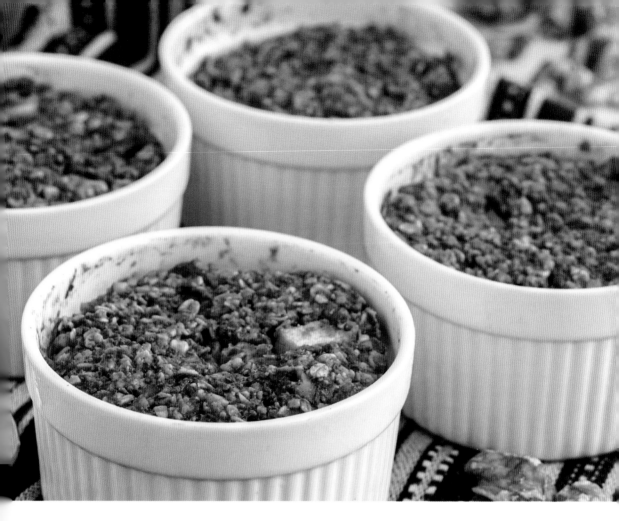

CHEF'S NOTES

Substitutions

Instead of a chia egg, use a flax egg
(1 tablespoon of flax meal to 3 tablespoons
of water).

In place of almond meal, use oat flour.

Use pears or other seasonal fruit of choice
in place of apple.

Keep It Nut Free

Simply omit the walnuts or substitute dried
fruit or pumpkin seeds for the walnuts.

Whole-Food Sweetener

Substitute date paste for coconut sugar,
but add it to the wet ingredients. Reduce
the amount of plant-based milk to ¾ cup.

Storage

Place leftovers in an airtight container in
the refrigerator for up to 3 days.

HARVEST GRAIN BREAKFAST BOWL

Breakfast bowls provide a delightful way to incorporate vegetables. They are effortless when you have the whole grains cooked and ready to go, and they will sustain you all morning long. Bonus: they are visually appealing, especially when you add an array of colorful plant-based foods. Treat the recipe below as a guide and feel free to make it your own by swapping out millet for another whole grain or substituting your favorite vegetables for the carrots, beets, or broccoli. Most importantly, have fun while experimenting!

Serves 4 **Prep time** 25 minutes **Cooking time** 30 minutes

Veggies

¾ cup carrots, diced
¾ cup beets, diced
1 cup broccoli florets
½ cup red onion, diced

Millet

1 cup dry organic millet
2 cups unsalted or low-sodium
   vegetable broth or water
¼ teaspoon salt, optional

Dressing

1 medium orange, peeled
   (see Chef's Notes)
1 tablespoon tahini
1 tablespoon apple cider vinegar
¼ teaspoon salt, optional
¼ cup fresh cilantro, roughly minced
   (optional)

Toppings

¼ cup unsweetened and unsulfured
   dried cranberries
¼ cup raw pumpkin seeds

1. Preheat the oven to 400°F. Line a baking sheet with parchment paper.
2. Boil 2 cups of water in a large stockpot. Add the carrots, beets, and broccoli, cooking for 5 to 7 minutes or until slightly tender.
3. Drain the stockpot and transfer the vegetables and red onion to the baking sheet. Roast for 25 minutes or until tender.
4. In a large, dry saucepan, toast the millet over medium heat for 4 to 5 minutes or until it turns a rich golden brown and becomes fragrant. Stir frequently to prevent burning.
5. Add 2 cups of vegetable broth or water to the millet and bring to a boil. Lower the heat to simmer, cover, and cook for 30 minutes. Let stand for 10 minutes before fluffing it with a fork.
6. In a food processor, puree all the dressing ingredients except the cilantro until smooth. Add the cilantro, pulse a few times, and set aside. If the dressing is too thick, add a bit of water as needed.
7. Divide the millet between two bowls and top with the roasted vegetables and dressing. Stir well and top with cranberries and pumpkin seeds.

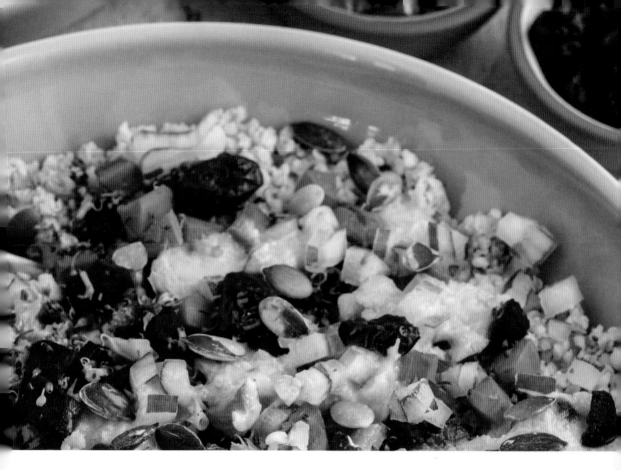

CHEF'S NOTES

Substitutions

Instead of millet, use quinoa, brown rice, or another organic whole grain of choice.

Substitute sweet potato or butternut squash for carrots.

Substitute cauliflower or brussels sprouts for broccoli.

Instead of roasted beets and carrots, try shredded raw beets and carrots.

Instead of cilantro, try chives or parsley.

Type of Orange

We used a juicy and seedless navel orange for the dressing. Using a sweet orange with no seeds would be ideal since you're blending the whole orange.

Prep Ahead

Prepare the millet ahead of time and store it in an airtight container in the refrigerator for up to 5 days (or freeze it for up to one month).

Prepare the dressing ahead of time and store it in the refrigerator for up to 5 days.

Prepare the roasted veggies ahead of time and store them in an airtight container in the refrigerator for up to 3 days.

Storage

Store leftovers in an airtight container in the refrigerator for up to 5 days or freeze them for up to one month.

COMFORTING CAULIFLOWER LENTIL KITCHARI

This is a house favorite at Food Revolution Network for its divine flavors, comforting warmth, and nourishing ingredients. Plus, it only takes ten minutes to prepare, and while it's cooking, your home will be filled with natural aromatherapy. The word *kitchari* means "mixture," and it's traditionally a combination of rice and mung beans in a warm soup-like dish, although a variety of grains and legumes can be used, like the lentils we use below. Bonus: If you want to eat more beans but fear the (gassy) consequences, kitchari is known for its digestive ease!

Serves 4 **Prep time** 10 minutes **Cooking time** 35 to 40 minutes

1 cup dry brown basmati rice, rinsed well

2 teaspoons mustard seeds

1 teaspoon cumin seeds

½ teaspoon fennel seeds

1 cup yellow onion, chopped

1 cup cauliflower florets, chopped into ½- to 1-inch pieces

1 tablespoon fresh ginger, grated

1 cup red lentils, rinsed well

1 teaspoon ground turmeric

¼ teaspoon ground coriander

4 cups unsalted or low-sodium vegetable broth

½ teaspoon salt, optional

¼ teaspoon ground black pepper, optional

1 to 2 tablespoons freshly squeezed lemon juice

Freshly chopped cilantro to taste, optional

Pinch crushed red pepper, optional

1. Boil 2 cups of water in a medium pot and heat on high until boiling. Add the rice and boil for 5 minutes.

2. Turn off the heat after 5 minutes and drain the rice. Set aside.

3. Heat a large pan on medium-high heat. Add the mustard, cumin, and fennel seeds and cook, stirring constantly, until the seeds begin to pop, about 2 minutes.

4. Reduce the heat to medium Add the onion, cauliflower, and ginger, and sauté for about 3 to 4 minutes, until the onion is tender and translucent. Deglaze the pan with water or vegetable broth as needed.

5. Stir in the rice, lentils, turmeric, coriander, vegetable broth, salt and pepper, and 2 cups of water. Bring to a boil over high heat. Lower the heat, cover, and simmer for 20 minutes.

6. Stir the kitchari well, and simmer, uncovered, for 10 to 15 minutes or until it resembles dal or soup. For a soupier texture, decrease the cooking time. For a thicker texture, cook it a bit longer. Taste and adjust the seasonings as desired.

7. Stir fresh lemon juice into the mixture and top with chopped cilantro and crushed red pepper, if desired.

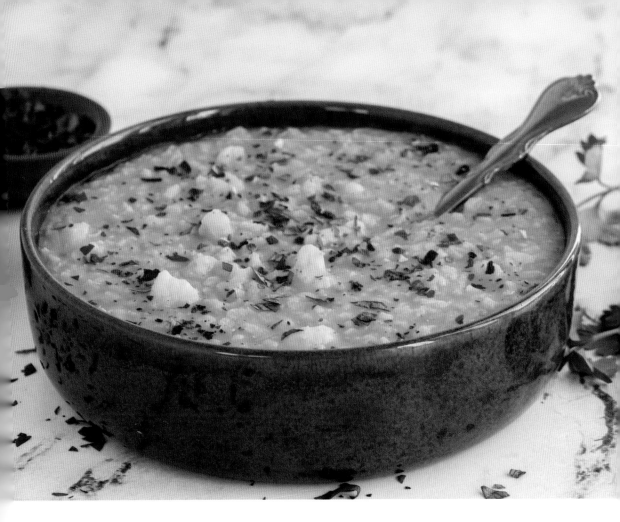

CHEF'S NOTES

Substitutions

Use any grain of choice, but make sure that the grain has the same cooking time as the lentils (about 20 to 30 minutes). If the grain requires a longer cooking time, precook it until al dente before adding it to the pan along with the lentils.

Instead of lentils, use mung beans.

In place of cauliflower, use broccoli, asparagus, carrots, or other vegetables of choice.

Add More Nutrition

Stir in chopped leafy greens before serving.

Add another vegetable when you add the cauliflower (such as carrots, peppers, or asparagus).

Storage

Store leftovers in an airtight container in the refrigerator for up to 5 days.

WARM BANANA CHIA BREAKFAST PUDDING

We included this pudding in the breakfast category because of its fiber, protein, and healthy fat composition from the chia seeds, oats, and walnuts. It could also easily fit into the dessert category—gently cooked bananas are something special!

Serves 2 **Prep time** 5 minutes **Cooking time** 10 minutes

Banana Topping

2 medium ripe bananas, sliced
2 tablespoons maple syrup
1 teaspoon vanilla extract
¼ teaspoon ground cinnamon
Pinch of ground nutmeg
Pinch of salt, optional

Pudding

2 cups unsweetened plant-based milk
⅓ cup chia seeds
½ cup rolled oats
1 teaspoon vanilla extract
Pinch of salt, optional
½ cup strawberries, sliced in half
¼ cup walnuts, chopped (optional)

1. Start the banana topping: Heat a medium pan on medium-high. Add the sliced bananas, stirring for 30 to 60 seconds.
2. Add the maple syrup, vanilla, cinnamon, nutmeg, and optional salt. Stir well so that the bananas are completely coated. Reduce the heat to medium-low and let the bananas cook for another 5 minutes, stirring occasionally. The bananas might start to get a little mushy, and that's okay! You'll want them soft and creamy. Set aside.
3. Make the chia pudding: Pour the milk into a medium saucepan. Stir in the chia, oats, vanilla, and optional salt. Heat the mixture over medium heat, continuously stirring until it has a pudding-like consistency (about 2 to 3 minutes).
4. Split the chia pudding between two bowls.
5. Mix in the bananas. Top with strawberries and walnuts.

CHEF'S NOTES

Substitutions

Instead of strawberries, use your fruit of choice, such as blueberries, raspberries, or kiwi.

In place of walnuts, use pecans or sliced almonds.

Whole-Food Sweetener

Use date paste in place of pure maple syrup.

Storage

Store leftovers in an airtight container in the refrigerator for up to 3 days. Chia seeds love to absorb liquids, so you may need to add more plant-based milk when you reheat this dish.

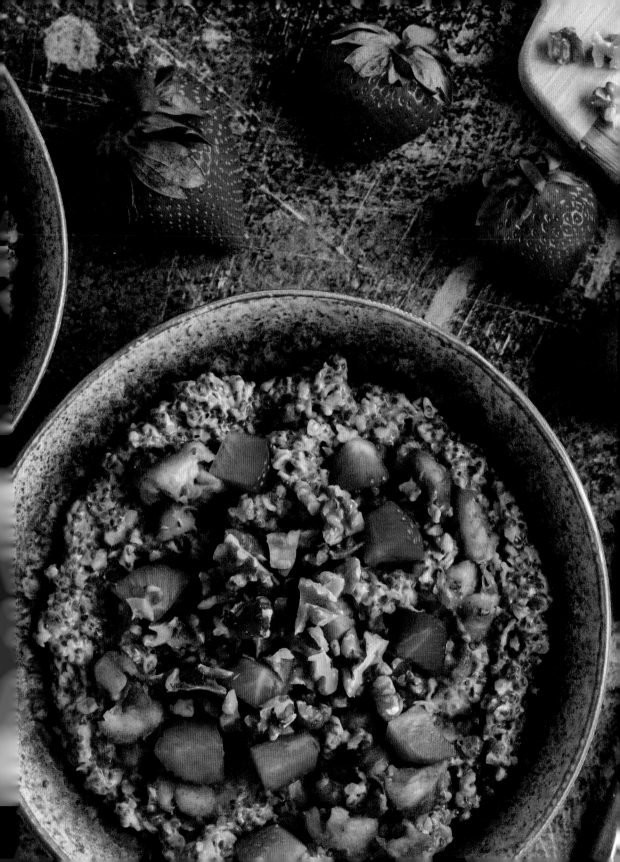

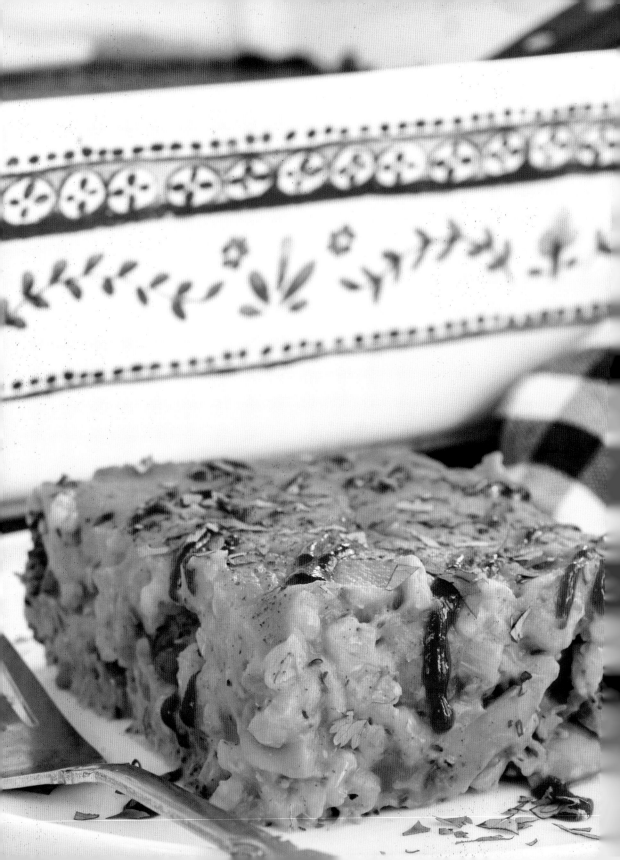

MOUTHWATERING MAINS

SIMPLE TRI-COLOR UMAMI STIR-FRY

Carrots, mushrooms, and spinach make a colorful feast for the eyes. This savory lunch or dinner has a hint of spice (feel free to omit it if it's not your thing) and aromatics that will make your kitchen smell warm and inviting. Serve this stir-fry with brown or black rice for a hearty meal that is bursting with flavor, color, and loads of veggies.

Serves 4 **Prep time** 15 minutes **Cooking time** 8 minutes

Sauce

1 tablespoon mellow yellow or chickpea miso

2 tablespoons reduced-sodium tamari or coconut aminos

2 tablespoons rice vinegar

1 tablespoon freshly squeezed lime juice

1 tablespoon maple syrup

1 teaspoon gochujang, sriracha, or chili paste, optional

¼ teaspoon garlic powder

¼ teaspoon ginger powder

2 teaspoons arrowroot powder

Stir-Fry

¼ cup unsalted or low-sodium vegetable broth

2 large carrots, spiralized or julienned (approximately 4 cups)

8 ounces mushrooms, chopped (approximately 3 cups)

4 medium garlic cloves, minced

2 cups spinach, chopped

1 cup frozen, shelled organic edamame

½ cup green onion, sliced

1. Whisk all the sauce ingredients in a medium bowl until the miso and arrowroot are dissolved. Set aside.

2. Heat a large pan on medium-high heat. Add the vegetable broth, carrots, and mushrooms. Cook until the carrots begin to soften, about 5 minutes, stirring occasionally.

3. Decrease the heat to medium and add the garlic. Cook for 1 minute. Add 1 to 2 tablespoons of water or vegetable broth as needed to deglaze the pan.

4. Stir in the spinach and edamame. Cook until the spinach is wilted, about 30 seconds.

5. Add the sauce, stirring until it thickens, about 30 to 60 seconds.

6. Transfer the stir-fry to a bowl and top with green onion.

7. When dividing the stir fry between plates, place on a bed of organic brown or black rice, if desired.

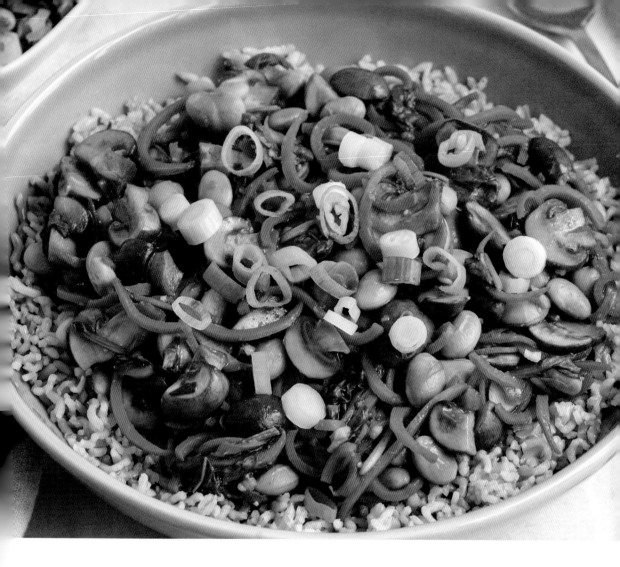

CHEF'S NOTES

Substitutions

For the mushrooms, use cremini, button, portobello, or other mushrooms of your choice.

Substitute other leafy greens of your choice in place of the spinach.

Instead of organic edamame, use chickpeas or other white beans of choice.

Whole-Food Sweetener

Use date paste in place of maple syrup.

Prep Ahead

Make the sauce ahead of time and store it in an airtight container in the refrigerator for up to 7 days.

Storage

Store leftovers in an airtight container in the refrigerator for up to 5 days.

PLANT-TASTIC MUSHROOM ZITI BAKE

Mushrooms take center stage in our superfood, plant-based spin on classic baked ziti. Not only do they make an ideal replacement when you're craving a meaty texture, but mushrooms also have plenty of fiber, vitamins, and phytonutrients that take this bake to the next level. It's perfect for a large family gathering or potluck and equally ideal for portioning away to enjoy as leftovers for lunch or dinner later in the week.

Serves 4 **Prep time** 25 minutes **Cooking time** 55 minutes

Tomato Sauce

1 28-ounce can plum tomatoes
1 cup yellow or white onion, chopped
5 garlic cloves, thinly sliced
2 cups mushrooms, sliced
¼ cup unsalted or low-sodium vegetable broth
15 ounces canned crushed tomatoes
1 teaspoon dried oregano
1 cup fresh basil, chopped
½ cup fresh parsley, chopped
¼ teaspoon salt, optional
2 cups spinach, chopped

Cashew Cheese

1 cup cashews, soaked (see Chef's Notes)
¼ cup nutritional yeast
2 tablespoons freshly squeezed lemon juice
1 teaspoon garlic powder
½ teaspoon salt, optional

Pasta

1 pound organic whole grain ziti (cook according to the directions on the package)

1. Preheat the oven to 350°F.
2. In a medium bowl, crush the whole plum tomatoes into smaller pieces and set aside. You'll combine these with the crushed tomatoes later.
3. In large skillet on medium-high heat, heat the onions, stir continuously, and cook until translucent, about 2 to 3 minutes.
4. Stir in the garlic and mushrooms. Deglaze the pan with veggie broth. Stir and cook for an additional 2 to 3 minutes.
5. Add both the plum tomatoes and can of crushed tomatoes to the skillet. Stir in the oregano, basil, parsley, and salt. Bring to a simmer for 15 minutes to thicken the sauce, stirring occasionally.
6. Add all the cheese ingredients with ½ cup of water to a blender or food processor and blend until smooth. Set aside.
7. Once the sauce has thickened, stir in the spinach and cook until tender.
8. Add half the cheese to the sauce and stir well.
9. Add the cooked pasta to the sauce, stir well, and then pour the mixture into a 9 x 13-inch baking dish. Dollop the remaining cheese on top of the ziti.
10. Bake for 30 minutes and let stand for 5 minutes before serving.

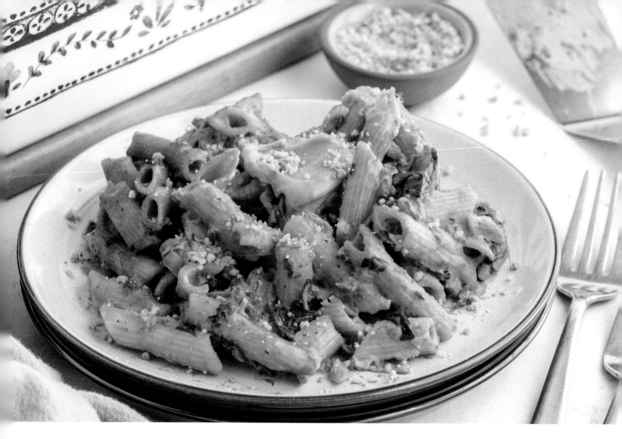

CHEF'S NOTES

Substitutions

Use shallots in place of onion.

For the mushrooms, use cremini, white button, portobello, or another mushroom of choice.

Instead of spinach, use another leafy green of choice.

Keep It Nut Free

Substitute raw sunflower seeds in place of cashews (they can be substituted in a 1:1 ratio).

Prep Ahead

Soak the cashews in hot water for 30 minutes or in room temperature water for 1 to 2 hours. Drain and rinse the cashews before adding them to the blender to make the cheese sauce.

Make the cashew cheese ahead of time and store it in an airtight container in the refrigerator for up to 3 days (or freeze it for up to 30 days and bring to the refrigerator for 24 hours before using it in the recipe).

Make the tomato sauce ahead of time and store it in an airtight container in the refrigerator for up to 3 days (or freeze it for up to 30 days).

Storage

Store leftovers in an airtight container in the refrigerator for up to 5 days.

BUILT TO GRILL BEANY MUSHROOM BURGERS

Veggie burgers get a bad rap for lacking flavor and being too crumbly to grill, which is a bummer because they can actually take on grillable textures and satisfying flavors. These mushroom burgers have a firm yet moist texture for the perfect chewy bite. Get ready to pile on the toppings (although this burger is bursting with flavor on its own) and experience a plant-based burger that truly hits the spot.

Serves 4 **Prep time** 20 minutes **Cooking time** 40 minutes

1 cup white or yellow onion, chopped

1½ cups button, portobello, or cremini mushrooms, chopped

2 tablespoons garlic, minced

1 tablespoon reduced-sodium tamari or coconut aminos

2 tablespoons vegan Worcestershire sauce

½ cup walnuts

¼ cup hulled hemp seeds

2 teaspoons onion powder

2 teaspoons smoked paprika

1½ cups home-cooked or canned white, great northern, cannellini, or navy beans, drained and rinsed

¾ cup oat flour

¼ cup fresh parsley, chopped (optional)

1. Preheat the oven to 400°F and line a baking sheet with parchment paper.

2. Sauté the veggies: Heat a large pan over medium-high heat. Add the onions and mushrooms, and cook for 3 to 4 minutes or until the onions are translucent.

3. Reduce the heat to medium and stir in the garlic. Cook for 1 minute. Add 1 to 2 tablespoons of water or vegetable broth to deglaze the pan as needed.

4. Stir in the tamari and Worcestershire sauce, and cook for an additional 1 to 2 minutes until the sauce is absorbed by the mushrooms. Remove the pan from the heat and set it aside.

5. Add the walnuts, hemp seeds, onion powder, and smoked paprika to a food processor and blend until a dough-like consistency is formed.

6. Add the onion and mushroom mixture to the walnuts and hemp, and pulse until the onions and mushrooms are mostly blended with the walnut-hemp mixture (some whole pieces are fine and preferred). Set aside.

7. In a large bowl, add the white beans and mash them with a potato masher or fork until ¾ of the beans are mashed and ¼ is left whole.

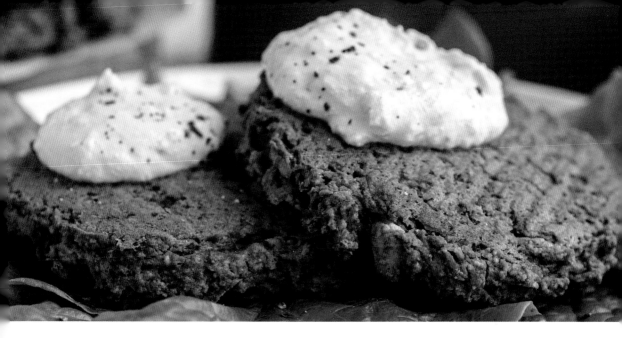

8. Transfer the mushroom-walnut mixture to the beans. Add the oat flour. Stir well until all ingredients are blended.

9. If using, stir in the parsley.

10. Scoop out a handful of the bean burger dough, form it into a patty, and place the patty on the lined baking sheet. Repeat with the remaining dough. You should have 6 to 8 patties.

11. Bake the patties for 30 minutes, flipping them halfway through.

12. Assemble the burger using your favorite bread, a whole grain wrap, or a lettuce wrap along with your favorite toppings!

CHEF'S NOTES

Substitutions

Instead of white or yellow onion, use red onion or shallots.

Instead of parsley, use basil, chives, or cilantro.

Keep It Nut Free

Use sunflower seeds in place of walnuts (they can be substituted in a 1:1 ratio).

Grilling Instructions

Place the burgers directly on a clean and slightly oiled grill over medium-high heat, cooking each side for 4 to 5 minutes until lightly browned.

Prep Ahead

Make the walnut-hemp mixture ahead of time and store it in an airtight container in the refrigerator for up to 5 days.

Storage

Store leftovers in an airtight container in the refrigerator for up to 5 days or in the freezer, separated by individual pieces of parchment paper, for up to 30 days.

AROMATIC VEGGIE-STUFFED ACORN SQUASH

Something about stuffed squash invites celebration, and what better way to celebrate our love of superfoods than with this wholesome dish! The delightful blend of sweet and savory brings out the best in each ingredient. Thanks to this dish's bright colors, varied textures, and diversity of spices, quinoa, lentils, and squash are finally getting the recognition they deserve. Each serving provides 41 grams of fiber and is packed with protein, carotenoids, and vitamin C. This dish makes for a satisfying dinner meal and is just as tasty (maybe even a bit better) as a leftovers lunch the next day.

Serves 2 **Prep time** 20 minutes **Cooking time** 50 minutes

Quinoa

½ cup dry organic quinoa
1 cup unsalted or low-sodium vegetable broth
1 pinch salt, optional

Acorn Squash

2 small acorn squash
2 pinches salt, optional
2 pinches ground black pepper, optional
1 tablespoon reduced-sodium tamari or coconut aminos
2 teaspoons maple syrup
½ tablespoon sherry vinegar or red wine vinegar

Filling

1 cup yellow onion, diced
¾ cup celery, diced
¾ cup red bell pepper, stemmed, seeded, and diced
1 cup mushrooms, diced
6 garlic cloves, minced
1 teaspoon ground turmeric
1 teaspoon ground cumin
1 teaspoon garam masala
½ teaspoon garlic powder
¼ teaspoon cinnamon
¼ cup unsalted or low-sodium vegetable broth
1 cup cooked lentils
¼ to ½ teaspoon salt, optional
Ground black pepper, to taste, optional
¼ cup unsweetened and unsulfured dried cranberries
¼ cup chopped pecans

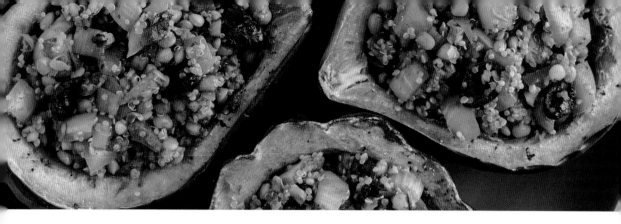

1. Add the quinoa, vegetable broth, and salt to a medium pot and bring to a boil. Reduce heat to a simmer, cover, and cook for 20 minutes. Set aside for 10 minutes, covered.

2. Preheat the oven to 375°F. Line a baking sheet with parchment paper.

3. Halve the squash and scoop out the seeds. Place it on the baking sheet, inner side up, and sprinkle with salt and pepper. Bake for 40 minutes.

4. Mix the tamari, maple syrup, and sherry vinegar in a small bowl. Once the squash halves are done baking, remove them from the oven (leaving the oven on) and brush the inside of each with the marinade. Set aside any remaining marinade. Bake the squash for an additional 10 minutes.

5. Heat a large pan on medium-high heat. Add the onions, celery, pepper, and mushrooms, continuously stirring until the onions are translucent, about 2 to 3 minutes.

6. Reduce the heat to medium, add the garlic, and cook for 30 to 60 seconds. Stir in the turmeric, cumin, garam masala, garlic powder, and cinnamon.

7. Deglaze the pan with ¼ cup of vegetable broth. Add the remaining squash marinade, if available. (It's not necessary, but adds a touch more flavor, so why waste it?)

8. Stir in the lentils, quinoa, and salt and pepper. Add the cranberries and pecans. Mix well and taste for seasoning.

9. Scoop even amounts of the quinoa/lentil mixture into each squash half. Serve by itself or with your favorite sauce or dressing (see notes).

CHEF'S NOTES

Substitutions

Use butternut or delicata squash in place of acorn squash.

Instead of quinoa, use organic brown rice or millet.

In place of red pepper, use green, yellow, or orange pepper.

Use mushrooms of your choice like portobello, button, cremini, or other mushrooms you love.

In place of lentils, use chickpeas, black beans, or another legume of choice.

Whole-Food Sweetener

Use date paste in place of maple syrup.

Creamy Sauces and Dressings

Top this recipe with a drizzle of tahini paste, your favorite plant-based dressing, or the Creamy Lemon Dijon Dressing from the Mighty Greens Power Bowl recipe on page 156.

Storage

Store leftovers in an airtight container in the refrigerator for up to 3 days.

MIGHTY GREENS POWER BOWL

Eating for health is never boring when you have the perfect combination of textures and flavors to excite your palate. If grain bowls are your plant-based go-to, then this bowl is sure to be a hit. Plus, it's super simple to make! Barley, broccolini, green beans, and snap peas make for a vibrant and nourishing bowl that has a variety of textures and flavors for a pleasant and unique grain bowl experience. Nutritionally speaking, this bowl is brimming with fiber from the barley and veggies, phytonutrients from the greens, and probiotics from the plant-based yogurt. You could also call this the gut-loving bowl!

Serves 2 **Prep time** 20 minutes **Cooking time** 10 minutes

Turmeric Barley

⅔ cup rinsed barley
½ teaspoon ground turmeric

Creamy Lemon Dijon Dressing

1 cup plain, unsweetened
  plant-based yogurt
1 tablespoon tahini
1 tablespoon Dijon mustard
¼ cup freshly squeezed lemon juice
2 tablespoons shallots, roughly
  chopped
1 tablespoon maple syrup
¼ teaspoon salt, optional

Mighty Greens

1 cup unsalted or low-sodium
  vegetable broth
5 garlic cloves, minced
3 cups (1 bunch) broccolini florets and
  stems, cut into 1-inch pieces
1 cup green beans, cut into 1-inch pieces
1 cup fresh or frozen green peas
Salt and ground black pepper to taste,
  optional
2 tablespoons sunflower seeds
Crushed red pepper to taste, optional

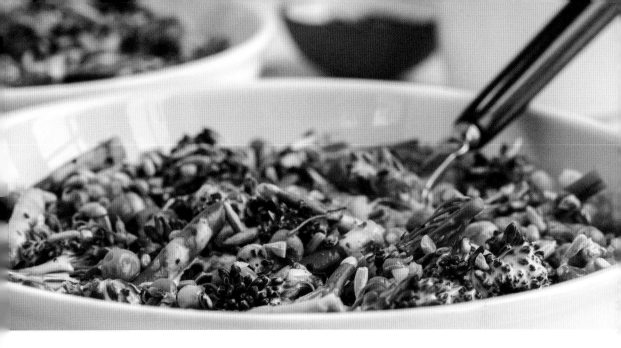

1. In a medium pot, bring the barley, 2 cups of water, turmeric, and black pepper to a boil. Reduce heat to a simmer, cover, and cook for at least 40 minutes. Taste test to check for tender barley (it'll be slightly chewy).

2. Blend all ingredients for the dressing in a blender or food processor until creamy. Taste and boost flavors as you desire (more lemon for acidity, more yogurt for tang, etc.) Set aside.

3. Add the vegetable broth, garlic, broccolini, green beans, and peas to a large pan. Add a sprinkle of salt and pepper. Heat over medium-high heat until boiling, then reduce the heat to a simmer and cover the pan with a lid ¾ of the way. Cook for 10 to 12 minutes or until the broccolini stems are tender.

4. If there is still liquid in the pan, remove the lid and continue cooking until most of the liquid is reduced.

5. Divide the barley between two serving bowls, then add the greens on top.

6. Drizzle with the desired amount of dressing, and sprinkle each bowl with a tablespoon of sunflower seeds and crushed red pepper.

CHEF'S NOTES

Substitutions

Use farro, wheat berries, or another whole grain of choice in place of barley.

Substitute cauliflower, regular broccoli, or brussels sprouts for broccolini.

Substitute edamame for green peas.

Gluten-Free Variation

Use quinoa, amaranth, millet, or brown rice in place of barley.

Prep Ahead

Cook the barley ahead of time and store it in an airtight container in the refrigerator for up to 5 days or freeze it for up to 30 days.

Make the Creamy Lemon Dijon Dressing ahead of time and store it in an airtight container in the refrigerator for up to 5 days.

Storage

Store leftovers in an airtight container in the refrigerator for up to 5 days.

PILE 'EM HIGH BLACK BEAN TOSTADAS

These tasty tostadas have lots of superfood power going for them. First, they're versatile—they can act as a satisfying main meal, fun appetizer, or sustaining snack. Second, they're packed with vitamins, minerals, and phytonutrients from the beans, sweet potatoes, and colorful slaw ingredients. Third, they're loaded with fiber and protein. Fourth, they allow you to practice your prep skills: the refried beans, slaw, and roasted veggies can all be made ahead of time so the meal is easy to assemble when you're hungry! This recipe is one of our favorites for many reasons, so we can't wait for you to try it.

Serves 4 **Prep time** 20 minutes **Cooking time** 40 minutes

Roasted Vegetables

¼ cup unsalted or low-sodium vegetable broth

1 teaspoon ground cumin

1 teaspoon onion powder

½ teaspoon chili powder

½ teaspoon salt, optional

2 cups sweet potatoes, diced, skin scrubbed and intact

2 cups poblano peppers, seeded and diced

Slaw Dressing

2 tablespoons tahini

¼ cup freshly squeezed lime juice

2 tablespoons organic rice vinegar

½ teaspoon salt, optional

Slaw Ingredients

3 cups purple cabbage, shredded

4 radishes, thinly sliced

1 cup red onion, diced

½ cup green onion, sliced

½ cup fresh cilantro, chopped (optional)

Other Ingredients

1½ cups home-cooked or canned refried black beans

4 organic whole grain or corn tortillas (5-inch to 8-inch)

1 large avocado, cubed

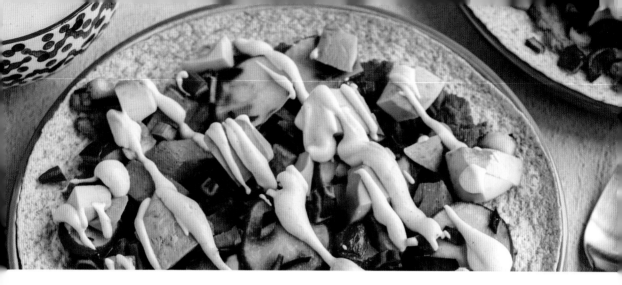

1. Preheat the oven to 400°F. Line a baking sheet with parchment.

2. Add the vegetable broth, cumin, onion powder, chili powder, and salt to a large bowl and mix well.

3. Add the sweet potatoes and poblano peppers to the bowl and toss well.

4. Transfer the vegetables to the baking sheet and roast for 25 minutes, tossing halfway through. Remove the veggies from the oven once they are tender and set aside. Leave the oven on but reduce the heat to 350°F.

5. While the veggies are cooking, whisk the tahini, lime juice, rice vinegar, and salt until the tahini is completely dissolved.

6. Add the cabbage, radishes, onions, and cilantro to the lime mixture and toss well. Set aside.

7. Place the tortillas on a pizza stone or baking sheet. Spread the refried beans evenly on each tortilla. Divide the roasted sweet potatoes and poblanos between the tortillas. Bake the tostadas for 10 to 15 minutes or until the tortillas are crispy.

8. Top each toastada with the cabbage, radish slaw, and avocado.

9. Serve with salsa and plant-based sour cream, if desired.

CHEF'S NOTES

Substitutions

Instead of poblano peppers, use red, orange, or yellow bell peppers.

In place of sweet potato, use purple or red potatoes.

In place of red onion for the slaw, use yellow or white onion.

Use pinto, kidney, or white beans in place of black beans.

Prep Ahead

Make the slaw ahead of time and store it in an airtight container in the refrigerator for up to 5 days.

If making home-cooked refried beans, make them ahead of time and store them in an airtight container in the refrigerator for up to 5 days or freeze for up to three months. If frozen, bring them to the refrigerator for 24 hours before using.

Make the vegetables ahead of time and store them in an airtight container in the refrigerator for up to 3 days.

Storage

Store the leftover slaw and vegetables separately in airtight containers in the refrigerator for up to 5 days.

NICE 'N' CHEESY COMFORTING CASSEROLE

We're pretty confident that you won't miss the dairy once you take a bite of this cheesy casserole. Cauliflower, butternut squash, and just the right amount of nutritional yeast create a remarkably umami and rich flavor that is the perfect complement to hearty pinto beans and broccoli. This casserole is comforting, nourishing, and sure to be a crowd favorite. Tip: Prepare the rice, beans, and cheese sauce ahead of time to help this dish come together easily and quickly!

Serves 6 **Prep time** 20 minutes **Cooking time** 30 minutes

Cauliflower Squash Cheese Sauce

1 cup yellow onion, chopped

3 garlic cloves, minced

3 cups fresh or frozen cauliflower florets, cut into 1-inch cubes

1 cup fresh or frozen butternut squash, cut into 1-inch cubes

1 teaspoon ground turmeric

¼ teaspoon ground black pepper, optional

1 cup unsalted or low-sodium vegetable broth

1 tablespoon organic mellow white or chickpea miso

3 tablespoons nutritional yeast

½ to 1 teaspoon smoked paprika

1 cup unsweetened plant-based milk

¼ to ½ teaspoon salt, optional

Casserole Filling

1½ cups onion, chopped

4 cups mushrooms, sliced

1 teaspoon dried oregano

¼ teaspoon salt, optional

¼ teaspoon ground black pepper, optional

3 cups broccoli florets, cut into 1-inch pieces

¼ cup unsalted or low-sodium vegetable broth

1½ cups home-cooked or canned pinto beans, drained and rinsed

4 cups cooked organic short-grain brown rice

⅓ cup jalapeño, diced, optional

2 tablespoons freshly squeezed lemon juice

½ to 1 teaspoon smoked paprika

Freshly chopped cilantro to taste, optional

Hot sauce of your choice to taste, optional

1. Make the Cauliflower Squash Cheese Sauce: Heat a large skillet over medium-high heat. Add the onions and cook until translucent, about 3 to 4 minutes. Add 1 to 2 tablespoons of water as needed to deglaze the pan.

2. Stir in the garlic and cook for another minute.

3. Stir in the cauliflower, squash, turmeric, and optional ground black pepper. Cook for an additional

minute before adding the vegetable broth. Turn the heat down to medium or to a simmer. Cover and cook for 7 to 10 minutes or until the cauliflower and squash are tender.

4. Remove from heat and transfer the cauliflower mixture to a blender or food processor (you may need to do this in two batches). Add the miso, nutritional yeast, smoked paprika, plant-based milk, and optional salt. Blend until smooth. Set aside.

5. Preheat the oven to 400°F and set your casserole dish aside.

6. Make the filling: Heat a large skillet over medium-high heat. Add the onions and mushrooms, cooking until the onions are translucent, about 3 to 5 minutes. Add 1 to 2 tablespoons of water as needed to deglaze the pan.

7. Stir in the oregano and optional salt and pepper, and cook for another minute.

8. Add the broccoli and vegetable broth (or water). Stir and cook until the veggie broth or water has evaporated, about 2 to 3 minutes (the broccoli will continue to cook in the oven).

9. Add the veggie filling, cooked rice, beans, optional jalapeños, and lemon juice to a large bowl. Stir to combine.

10. Add one cup of the Cauliflower Squash Cheese Sauce to the bowl and stir well.

11. Transfer the mixture to a casserole dish, spreading out evenly.

12. Pour the remaining sauce over top of the casserole. Sprinkle with more smoked paprika, if desired.

13. Bake for 30 minutes or until golden brown on top. Let the casserole set for 10 to 15 minutes before serving.

14. Divide between plates and top with chopped cilantro and hot sauce, if desired.

CHEF'S NOTES

Substitutions

Use white onion in place of yellow onion.

Use sweet paprika in place of smoked paprika (however, note that you'll lose the smoky flavor).

Substitute wild rice, red rice, or black rice for brown rice.

Substitute black beans, kidney beans, or other beans of choice for the pinto beans.

For the mushrooms, use cremini, portobello, or button mushrooms.

Use cauliflower in place of broccoli.

Use serrano peppers in place of jalapeños.

Prep Ahead

Make the rice ahead of time and store it in an airtight container in the refrigerator for up to 3 days before making this recipe (or freeze it for up to one month).

Make your beans ahead of time if you're making home-cooked, and store them in an airtight container in the refrigerator for up to 3 days before making this recipe (or freeze them for up to one month).

Make the Cauliflower Squash Cheese Sauce ahead of time and store it in an airtight container in the refrigerator for up to 3 days before making this recipe.

Storage

Store veggie casserole leftovers in an airtight container in the refrigerator for up to 5 days or freeze them for up to one month.

Store cheese sauce leftovers in an airtight container in the refrigerator for up to 5 days or freeze them for up to one month.

SOUTH OF THE BORDER BLACK BEAN BURGERS

One way to ensure healthy eating is by preparing easy and versatile meals. Feast on this Mexican-inspired burger by placing it between a whole grain bun with veggies piled high (leafy greens, tomato, onion, and sprouts are all great options) or crumble it as a filling for tacos. You could also swap out the whole grain bread with collard greens to make a vibrant veggie wrap. The simplicity of this recipe and the variety of ways to enjoy these burgers make it a plant-based meal that is convenient, delicious, and nutritious.

Serves 6 **Prep time** 20 minutes **Cooking time** 40 minutes

¾ cup onion, diced

½ cup red bell pepper, stemmed, seeded, and diced

3 garlic cloves, minced

1 to 2 jalapeños, seeded and minced, optional

¾ cup fresh or frozen organic corn

1 teaspoon dried oregano

1½ cups home-cooked or canned black beans, drained and rinsed

½ cup oat flour or almond meal

2 to 4 tablespoons flax meal

1 tablespoon cumin

1 tablespoon chili powder

1 tablespoon onion powder

1 teaspoon garlic powder

¼ cup fresh cilantro, chopped, optional

1 tablespoon freshly squeezed lime juice

½ teaspoon salt, optional

¼ teaspoon ground black pepper, optional

Red pepper flakes to taste, optional

1. Preheat the oven to 400°F and line a baking sheet with parchment paper.

2. In a large skillet over medium-high heat, add the onions and red peppers, stirring often, until the onions are translucent, about 2 to 3 minutes. Add 1 to 2 tablespoons of water as needed to deglaze the pan.

3. Turn the heat down to medium and stir in the garlic, jalapeño, corn, and oregano. Cook for an additional 2 to 3 minutes before setting aside.

4. Add the black beans to a large bowl and mash until ¾ are mashed and ¼ is whole (for texture).

5. In a separate bowl, combine the oat flour (or almond meal), 2 tablespoons of flax meal, cumin, chili powder, onion powder, garlic powder, cilantro, and lime juice.

6. Stir the corn mixture into the bean mixture until combined. Add salt and black pepper to taste.

7. If the mixture doesn't hold together when you try to form a patty, add an additional 1 to 2 tablespoons of flax meal until you reach a moist dough consistency.

8. Scoop a handful of the bean burger dough into your hand, form into a patty, and place on the baking sheet. Repeat until you have 6 to 8 patties.

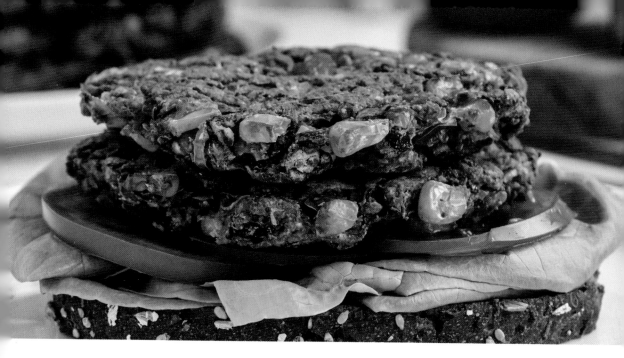

9. Bake for 40 minutes, flipping halfway through. Alternatively, grill the burgers until each side is golden brown, about 5 to 7 minutes per side.

CHEF'S NOTES

Substitutions

Substitute white beans, kidney beans, or pinto beans for black beans.

Instead of red bell pepper, use orange or yellow bell pepper.

For the onion, use white, yellow, or red.

Substitute whole wheat flour in place of oat flour.

Instead of cilantro, use parsley or chives.

Serving Options

Make a traditional burger or sandwich with a whole grain bun or bread and lots of veggies like leafy greens, tomato, and sprouts.

Crumble the cooked patties and add them to a taco or burrito or to casseroles and grain bowls.

Make a wrap with collard greens and crunchy veggies (carrot, celery, or cucumber).

Add to a salad as your "protein."

Prep Ahead

If using home-cooked beans, store them in an airtight container in the refrigerator for up to 3 days before making the recipe (or freeze cooked beans for up to 3 months and thaw before using).

Storage

Store leftovers in an airtight container in the refrigerator for up to 5 days or in the freezer, separated by individual pieces of parchment paper, for up to 30 days.

SPROUT AND FLOURISH GRAIN BOWL

This bowl has all the elements of a superfood meal: plenty of fiber, vitamins, minerals, and phytonutrients, as well as the perfect balance of plant-based fat, protein, and carbohydrates to keep you satisfied and nourished. Drizzle with our decadent creamy garlic sauce and top with alfalfa sprouts (or your favorite sprouts) for a restaurant-quality meal made right in your own home!

Serves 2 **Prep time** 20 minutes **Cooking time** none

Garlic Sauce

1 cup cashews, soaked in hot water for 30 minutes or room temperature water for 1 to 2 hours, drained

2 teaspoons garlic powder

½ teaspoon mustard powder

½ teaspoon onion powder

2 teaspoons mellow white or chickpea miso

¼ teaspoon salt, optional

2 tablespoons jalapeño, seeded and chopped, optional

Bowl Ingredients

4 cups mixed greens

1 cup cooked quinoa (see Chef's Notes)

1 cup cooked bean sprouts (see Chef's Notes)

1 large avocado, cubed

1 cup cucumber, sliced (peel if the skin is waxed)

1 cup carrot, shredded

1 cup alfalfa sprouts

1. Drain the soaked cashews and place them in a food processor or blender.

2. Add the remaining garlic sauce ingredients to a cup of water and blend until smooth.

3. Assemble the bowl ingredients: In two separate bowls, first add the cooked quinoa followed by the cooked bean sprouts, avocado, cucumber, and carrot.

4. Pour your desired amount of garlic sauce over the top and mix it together with the bowl ingredients.

5. Divide the alfalfa sprouts between bowls and enjoy!

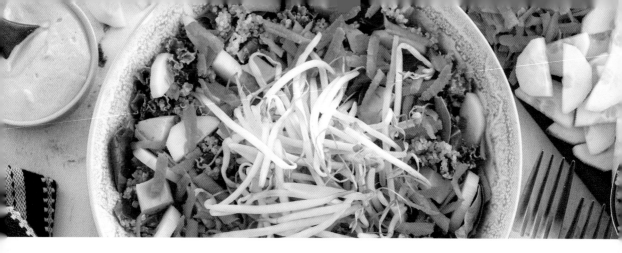

CHEF'S NOTES

Substitutions

Any vegetables lounging around your kitchen are great for grain bowls!

In place of quinoa, try organic brown rice, farro, wheat berries, or sweet potato.

Cook the Quinoa

Add ⅓ cup dry quinoa (but well rinsed) and ⅔ cup water to a stovetop pot. Bring to a boil, then lower to a simmer, cover, and cook for 15 minutes. Remove from heat and allow to sit, covered, for 10 minutes before fluffing with a fork.

Layer It Up

The options here are endless! Top the bowl with herbs like dill, cilantro, basil, or oregano.

Add additional protein like grilled tempeh or tofu, lentils, or seeds.

Sprinkle with chia, hemp, or flaxseeds for a nutritional crunch.

Sprinkle with nutritional yeast for some cheesiness.

About Sprouts

Feel free to choose any sprouts you love—broccoli, clover, and sunflower all come to mind. Note that bean sprouts should always be cooked for digestibility. Because of the risk that comes with eating sprouts, children, pregnant women, the elderly, and people with generally weaker immune systems are encouraged to thoroughly cook sprouts—especially if they come from a store. Cook bean sprouts in a steamer basket for 15 minutes or sauté with ¼ cup of water over medium-high heat until slightly tender and the water has evaporated.

Keep It Nut Free

Use sunflower seeds in place of cashews in a 1:1 ratio.

Prep Ahead

Store the quinoa in an airtight container for up to 5 days in the refrigerator or three months in the freezer.

Cook the bean sprouts ahead of time and store them in an airtight container for up to 2 days.

Garlic Sauce Uses

Thin out leftover garlic sauce with a bit of water to make a delicious salad dressing or keep it as is to pour over baked sweet potatoes or a pasta dish.

Storage

Store the sauce in an airtight container in the refrigerator for up to 5 days or freeze for up to one month. Store the bowl ingredients in an airtight container in the refrigerator for up to 2 days.

HARISSA-SPICED CAULIFLOWER AND CHICKPEAS WITH COOLING CUCUMBER YOGURT

Harissa is a North African spice blend that incorporates ground chilies, garlic, coriander seeds, caraway seeds, and cumin seeds. This complex blend of herbs and spices adds a robust and uniquely smoky flavor to many dishes—in this case, cauliflower and chickpeas. Serve this delightful, smoky-cool combination on top of cooked bulgur with a hint of squeezed lemon for a dish that will make your taste buds sing.

Serves 4 **Prep time** 20 minutes **Cooking time** 30 minutes

Cauliflower

1 small head cauliflower, chopped into 1- to 2-inch florets (approximately 6 cups)

1½ cups home-cooked or canned chickpeas, drained and rinsed

1 tablespoon avocado oil, optional

2 tablespoons harissa spice blend

2 to 3 pinches of salt, optional

Pickled Red Onions

1 small red onion, thinly sliced

½ cup red wine vinegar

¼ teaspoon salt, optional

Cucumber Yogurt

1 cup plain, unsweetened plant-based yogurt

1 cup cucumber, peeled, grated, and water removed (see Chef's Notes)

1 tablespoon red, yellow, or white onion, grated

¼ cup fresh cilantro, chopped, optional

2 teaspoons apple cider vinegar

1 teaspoon ground cumin

¼ teaspoon salt, optional

¼ teaspoon ground black pepper, optional

Other Bowl Ingredients

3 cups cooked bulgur

¼ cup fresh parsley, minced

4 lemon wedges

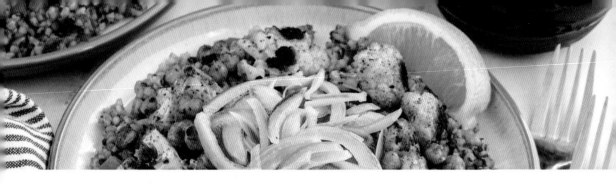

1. Preheat the oven to 425°F and line a baking sheet with parchment paper.
2. In a large bowl, mix together the cauliflower, chickpeas, optional avocado oil, harissa spice blend, and optional salt. Stir until the cauliflower and chickpeas are well coated.
3. Spread them out evenly on the parchment-lined baking sheet and roast for 30 minutes, tossing halfway through.
4. Meanwhile, make the pickled onions: Slice the onions thin with a mandoline or manually with a chef's knife.
5. Add the sliced onions, red wine vinegar, ½ cup of water, and optional salt to a large bowl. Massage the onions into the red wine vinegar. Set aside.
6. Next, make the cucumber yogurt: Mix all the ingredients together in a medium bowl and set aside.
7. Divide the cooked bulgur between four plates or bowls.
8. Once the cauliflower and chickpeas are done roasting, divide them between the bowls.
9. Top each bowl with 2 to 3 forkfuls of pickled onions. Sprinkle with parsley and serve with lemon wedges.
10. Serve the cucumber yogurt alongside the dish or add 2 to 4 spoonfuls on top of each bowl.

CHEF'S NOTES

Substitutions

Substitute broccoli or brussels sprouts for cauliflower.

Instead of chickpeas, use another white bean of choice.

For the onion, use yellow, white, or red.

Substitute parsley, chives, or dill for cilantro.

Preparing the Cucumber

After grating the cucumber, grab a handful and squeeze it to release as much water as possible. Set that cucumber aside in a bowl and move on to the next handful. Do this until you've squeezed as much water as possible out of all the cucumber.

Gluten-Free Variation

Substitute quinoa, millet, or brown rice for bulgur.

Prep Ahead

Cook the bulgur ahead of time and store it in an airtight container in the refrigerator for up to 5 days or in the freezer for up to one month.

Make the Pickled Red Onions ahead of time and store them in an airtight container in the refrigerator for up to 10 days.

Make the cucumber yogurt ahead of time and store it in an airtight container in the refrigerator for up to 5 days.

Storage

Store leftovers in an airtight container in the refrigerator for up to 5 days.

(BRING LA) FIESTA ROASTED SWEET POTATO BOWL

Energizing and healing spices combined with fiber-rich lentils and corn, phytonutrient superstar kale, and a nutrient-packed array of toppings—this hearty bowl will leave you doing a happy dance! Roasted sweet potatoes tossed in zesty herbs and spices then piled high with purple cabbage, lentils, corn, avocado, and pickled red onions is a feast for both your eyes and palate. Once you give this recipe a try, you'll understand why this bowl ranks as one of our favorites!

Serves 4 **Prep time** 15 minutes **Cooking time** 30 minutes

4 cups sweet potatoes, scrubbed and cut into 1-inch cubes

Fiesta Seasoning

½ teaspoon onion powder
½ teaspoon garlic powder
½ teaspoon paprika
¼ teaspoon chili powder
1 teaspoon ground cumin
¼ teaspoon salt, optional
¼ teaspoon ground black pepper, optional

Coconut Tahini Dressing

½ cup light coconut milk
1 tablespoon tahini
1 tablespoon freshly squeezed lime juice
¼ teaspoon garlic powder
¼ teaspoon salt, optional

Lentils and Corn

2 cups cooked brown or green lentils
2 cups cooked fresh or frozen organic corn
2 tablespoons freshly squeezed lime juice

Kale

4 cups organic kale, stemmed and chopped
2 tablespoons freshly squeezed lemon juice
Pinch of salt to taste, optional

Toppings

2 to 3 forkfuls Pickled Red Onions (see page 166 for recipe)
½ cup purple cabbage, shredded
2 to 4 tablespoons jalapeño, seeded and chopped, optional
1 large avocado, cubed
2 to 4 tablespoons fresh cilantro, chopped, optional

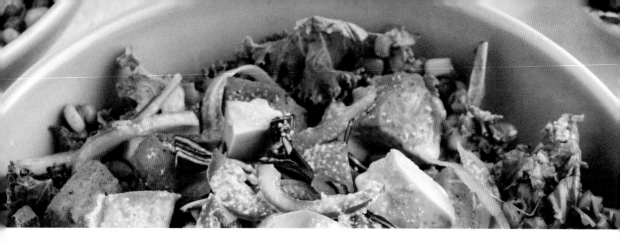

1. Preheat the oven to 400°F and line a baking sheet with parchment paper.
2. Mix the seasoning ingredients together in a small bowl.
3. In a large bowl, toss the sweet potatoes with half the seasoning.
4. Spread the sweet potatoes out evenly on the baking sheet and bake for 30 minutes, flipping halfway through.
5. Meanwhile, in a mason jar or medium bowl, add the coconut milk, tahini, lime juice, and garlic powder. Place the lid on the mason jar and shake well or stir well in a bowl until all of the tahini is dissolved. Set aside.
6. In a large bowl, mix the lentils and corn with the lime juice and remaining seasoning blend. Set aside.
7. In a large bowl, massage the kale with the lemon juice and a sprinkle of salt until soft, about 30 seconds.
8. Split the kale, lentil and corn mixture, and sweet potatoes between four bowls.
9. Add a few forkfuls of the pickled onions to each bowl.
10. Sprinkle cabbage, jalapeño, and avocado, and 1 to 2 tablespoons of coconut tahini dressing on top. Sprinkle with cilantro, if desired.

CHEF'S NOTES

Substitutions

Instead of sweet potatoes, use purple or red potatoes.

Use butternut squash in place of sweet potato.

Instead of lentils, use your favorite legume.

Substitute your favorite leafy green for kale.

Use unsweetened plant-based yogurt in place of coconut milk for the dressing.

Cooking the Lentils

Thoroughly rinse 1 cup dry lentils and boil in 3 cups of water. Then lower to a simmer, cover, and cook for 20 to 25 minutes. This will yield approximately 2½ cups of cooked lentils.

Prep Ahead

Cook the lentils and corn ahead of time. Store them separately in airtight containers in the refrigerator for up to 5 days or freeze for up to 3 months.

Make the Pickled Red Onions ahead of time.

Make the Coconut Tahini Dressing ahead of time and store it in an airtight container in the refrigerator for up to 5 days.

Storage

Store leftovers in an airtight container in the refrigerator for up to 3 days.

EVERYDAY LENTIL LUNCH

This tasty lunch dish got its name for a reason. Lentils, brown rice, veggies, nuts, and seeds come together for a meal that is ready in minutes. Mushrooms and bok choy taste delicious here, but you can use any veggies you have on hand or that you prefer. Cook up extra lentils and brown rice to prepare for when the craving hits, as this could become your new go-to lunch every day of the week.

Serves 4 **Prep time** 10 minutes **Cooking time** 10 minutes

1 teaspoon mustard seed

1 teaspoon cumin seed

1 bunch bok choy, stems chopped, leaves sliced and separated (see Chef's Notes)

2 cups mushrooms, sliced

½ cup unsalted or low-sodium vegetable broth

3 medium-large garlic cloves, minced

1 tablespoon fresh ginger, minced

1 teaspoon ground turmeric

1½ teaspoons ground cumin

¼ teaspoon salt, optional

¼ teaspoon ground black pepper, optional

2 cups cooked brown or green lentils

2 cups cooked organic brown or black rice

1 to 2 tablespoons freshly squeezed lime juice

1 to 2 green onion stalks, sliced

¼ cup cashews or sunflower seeds

¼ cup fresh cilantro, chopped, optional

Crushed red pepper to taste, optional

1. In a medium saucepan, toast the mustard and cumin seeds on medium heat until fragrant or they start to "pop," about 2 minutes.

2. Add the bok choy stems (reserve the leaves for later) and mushrooms. Cook for 2 minutes, stirring occasionally to prevent them from sticking.

3. Add ¼ cup of vegetable broth to deglaze the pan and continue cooking for another 3 minutes, stirring occasionally.

4. Add the garlic, ginger, ground turmeric, ground cumin, and optional salt and pepper. Cook for an additional 1 to 2 minutes.

5. Add the lentils and rice plus the other ¼ cup of vegetable broth. Stir and cook until the broth is absorbed and lentils and rice are warmed through.

6. Remove from the heat. Stir in the bok choy leaves until they are tender and squeeze in the lime juice.

7. Divide between plates and sprinkle with green onion, cashews, and optional cilantro and crushed red pepper.

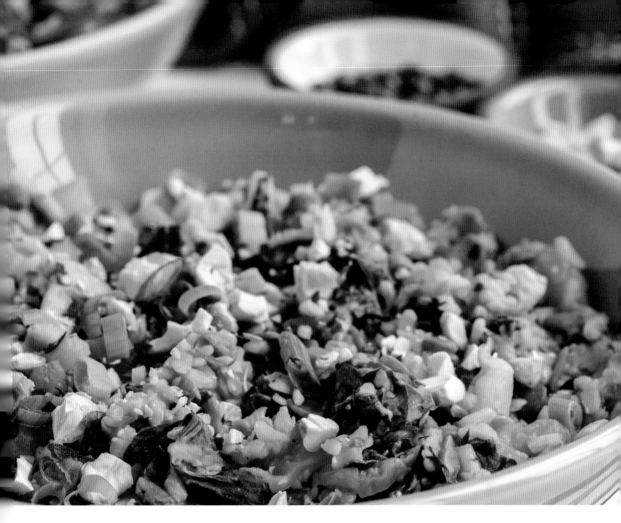

CHEF'S NOTES

Substitutions

Instead of lentils, use another legume like chickpeas, black beans, or edamame.

Instead of rice, try quinoa, millet, farro, or wheat berries.

Use any kind of mushroom you love like shiitake, button, or portobello.

Substitute lemon juice for lime juice.

Use another herb in place of cilantro, such as parsley, basil, or chives.

Bok Choy

You can use a different leafy green. If you only use leafy greens (and not the stems) add them at the end where you would add the bok choy leaves.

Prep Ahead

Make the lentils and rice ahead of time and store them in an airtight container in the refrigerator for up to 3 days.

Storage

Store leftovers in an airtight container in the refrigerator for up to 5 days.

KICKIN' KIMCHI "FRIED" RICE AND VEGGIES

Fermented make your gut microbiome happy, which is why we consider them to be superfoods. Our sautéed, not-fried, version includes traditional (brown) rice and fermented kimchi (great for your gut health) along with plenty of broccoli, carrots, peppers, and snap peas. Topped with nuts and seeds, it also offers healthy plant-based fat, protein, lots of phytonutrients, and some deliciously satisfying crunch.

Serves 4 **Prep time** 20 minutes **Cooking time** 15 minutes

1 cup onion, diced

1 cup red bell pepper, stemmed, seeded, and diced

1 cup carrots, diced

6 garlic cloves, minced

1 tablespoon fresh ginger, minced

2 cups broccoli florets, cut into 1-inch pieces

1 cup snap peas

2 tablespoons reduced-sodium tamari or coconut aminos

1 tablespoon umeboshi plum vinegar or red wine vinegar

4 cups cooked organic brown rice

1 cup kimchi, chopped (see Chef's Notes)

2 tablespoons black or white sesame seeds

2 tablespoons green onion, sliced

⅓ cup cashews, chopped, optional

1 teaspoon sesame oil, optional

2 tablespoons fresh cilantro, chopped, optional

1. Sauté your veggies: Heat a large pot on medium-high heat. Add the onions, peppers, and carrots. Cook until the onions are translucent and the carrots are tender, about 5 to 7 minutes. Add 1 to 2 tablespoons of water or vegetable broth as needed to deglaze the pan.

2. Turn the heat down to medium and stir in the garlic, ginger, broccoli, and snap peas. Cook for an additional 3 to 4 minutes. Again, deglaze the pan with water or vegetable broth as needed.

3. Stir in the tamari and vinegar and cook for another 1 to 2 minutes.

4. Add the rice and kimchi. Stir until combined with the vegetables.

5. Remove the pot from the heat and stir in the sesame seeds, green onion, and optional cashews, sesame oil, and cilantro.

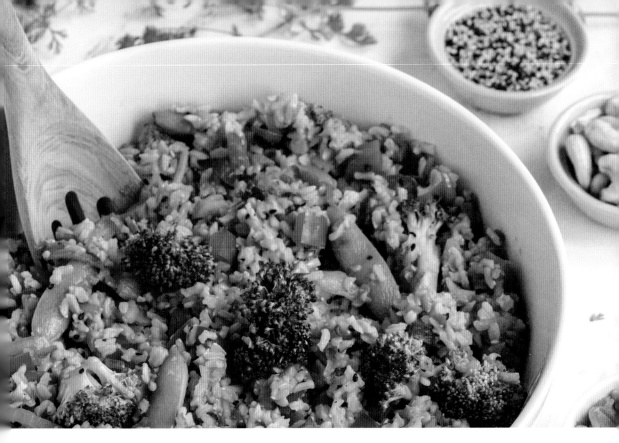

CHEF'S NOTES

Substitutions

For the onion, use white or yellow onion or shallots.

Substitute yellow, orange, or green bell pepper for red pepper.

Instead of broccoli, use broccolini or cauliflower.

Substitute snow peas for snap peas.

Instead of brown rice, use another whole grain of choice.

Kimchi

You can make your own, but store-bought is also a great option. You can use radish or cabbage kimchi; just make sure that the package states "live culture" or "with probiotics," and that it's not pasteurized (since pasteurization kills the friendly bacteria). This will ensure you get all of the probiotic benefits.

Prep Ahead

Cut the onion, pepper, carrots, and broccoli ahead of time and store them in an airtight container in the refrigerator for up to 2 days before preparing the meal.

Storage

Store leftovers in an airtight container in the refrigerator for up to 5 days or freeze them for up to 30 days.

VEGGED-OUT TOFU PAD THAI

This big bowl of noodles is as nourishing as it is comforting. Tofu is packed with plant-based protein, carrots and peppers have lots of carotenoids, and garlic offers prebiotic fiber. This dish is filled with a rainbow of colors, a symphony of flavors, and a variety of textures that are nourishing for your body and soul.

Serves 2 **Prep time** 20 minutes **Cooking time** 40 minutes

Tofu

¼ cup cornmeal
¼ cup oat flour or almond flour
1 teaspoon garlic powder
1 teaspoon onion powder
½ teaspoon salt, optional
14 ounces firm or extra firm tofu, drained and pressed, cut into 1-inch cubes

Pad Thai Sauce

3 tablespoons tomato paste
4 tablespoons reduced-sodium tamari or coconut aminos
3 tablespoons maple syrup
¼ cup freshly squeezed lime juice
1 tablespoon chili paste, optional
2 tablespoons mellow white or chickpea miso

Noodles

8 ounces pad thai noodles, dry

Vegetables

1 large carrot, julienned
1 medium red bell pepper, stemmed, seeded, and julienned
2 garlic cloves, minced
1 cup mung bean sprouts
2 to 3 green onion stalks, both green and white parts, sliced
¼ cup fresh cilantro, chopped, optional
¼ cup raw or roasted peanuts
Lime wedges for serving

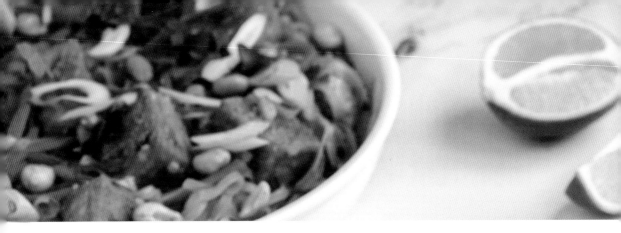

1. Preheat the oven to 400°F. Line a baking sheet with parchment paper.
2. Add the cornmeal, oat flour, garlic powder, onion powder, and salt to a large bowl. Add the tofu and toss gently to coat. If the tofu is too soft, coat each piece individually, then transfer to the baking sheet.
3. Bake for 40 minutes, tossing halfway through.
4. Meanwhile, whisk all the sauce ingredients along with 6 tablespoons of water in a medium bowl until the miso is dissolved. Alternatively, you can mix the sauce in a blender. Set aside.
5. Make the noodles as instructed. Set aside. Heat a wok or large pan over medium-high heat. Add the carrots and red peppers, cooking until the carrots are tender, about 5 to 7 minutes, stirring occasionally. If they stick to the pan, add a few tablespoons of water or vegetable broth.
6. Stir in the garlic and cook for 30 to 60 seconds. Stir in the mung bean sprouts and noodles. Then add the tofu and sauce. Stir until the noodles, tofu, and vegetables are fully mixed with the sauce.
7. Top with green onions, peanuts, and cilantro. Serve with lime wedges.

CHEF'S NOTES

Substitutions

Instead of tofu, add frozen, shelled edamame.

In place of red pepper, use orange, yellow, or green bell pepper.

Instead of mung bean sprouts, use sunflower sprouts or snow peas.

In place of cilantro, use basil or parsley.

Keep It Nut Free

Omit the peanuts or use sunflower seeds instead.

Whole-Food Sweetener

Use date paste in place of maple syrup.

Prep Ahead

Prepare the tofu ahead of time and store it in an airtight container in the refrigerator for up to 3 days. (Reheat in the oven at 400°F for 10 to 15 minutes before adding to the noodles.)

Make the sauce ahead of time and store it in an airtight container in the refrigerator for up to 5 days.

Cut the vegetables ahead of time and store them in an airtight container in the refrigerator for up to 3 days.

Storage

Store leftovers in an airtight container in the refrigerator for up to 5 days.

EVERYTHING BUT THE KITCHEN SINK POTATO NACHOS

Are nachos a superfood? Traditional nachos, not so much. These loaded potato nachos? Absolutely! This dish is not only tasty but bursting with a wide variety of phytonutrients from every color of the rainbow. Plus, these yummy nachos are a great opportunity to get family members involved with adding their favorite tasty and nutritious toppings.

Serves 2 to 4 **Prep time** 20 minutes **Cooking time** 30 minutes

Spice Mixture

1½ teaspoons chili powder
1½ teaspoons onion powder
1 teaspoon garlic powder
1 teaspoon smoked paprika, optional
¼ cup nutritional yeast
½ teaspoon salt, optional

Potatoes

2 pounds organic potatoes, cut into ¼-inch-thick rounds

Cilantro Cream (optional)

8 ounces firm tofu
¾ cup fresh cilantro, chopped
½ cup freshly squeezed lime juice

¼ cup jalapeños, seeded and chopped, optional
1 teaspoon ground cumin
¼ teaspoon salt, optional

Toppings

1½ cups spinach, chopped
¾ cup tomatoes, diced
1 cup home-cooked or canned black beans, drained and rinsed
1 cup canned or frozen organic corn
¼ cup red onion, diced
¼ cup black olives, diced
2 to 4 tablespoons jalapeños, seeded and sliced, optional
1 large avocado, seeded and cubed
¼ cup fresh cilantro, chopped, optional
Hot sauce to taste, optional

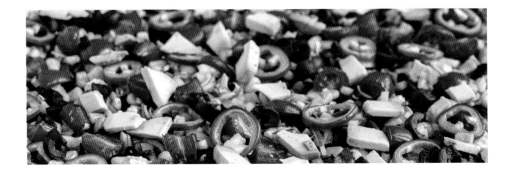

1. Preheat the oven to 400°F. Line a large baking sheet with parchment paper.

2. Prepare your potato spice mix: In a medium bowl, mix all of the spice ingredients together until blended.

3. Dip each potato slice into the spice mix to coat each side of the potato. Spread out the potatoes evenly on the baking sheet. (The natural moisture of the potatoes will help the spice mix to stick. However, if it doesn't stick, brush the potatoes lightly with vegetable broth or water, then dip into the spice mixture.)

4. Bake the potatoes for 20 minutes, flipping halfway through.

5. While the potatoes are baking, prepare the Cilantro Cream, if using. Add all ingredients to a food processor and blend until creamy. Alternatively, you could use an immersion blender, blending until the tofu is creamy and most of the cilantro is blended.

6. Taste and boost the flavors of your choice (more jalapeño for spice, more lime juice for tartness, or more cilantro for an earthy flavor). For a thinner consistency, add 1 to 2 tablespoons of water at a time until it thins out satisfactorily.

7. Once the potatoes are finished cooking, line them up close together on the baking sheet so gaps are minimal (in preparation for adding the toppings).

8. Add a layer of spinach across the potatoes. Then add the tomatoes, beans, corn, red onion, black olives, and optional jalapeños.

9. Bake for 10 minutes, then remove the sheet from the oven and add the avocado and optional cilantro.

10. Finally, if you'd like to add a little creaminess, drizzle the Cilantro Cream on top. Add your favorite hot sauce for an added kick!

CHEF'S NOTES

Substitutions

We used russet potatoes, but red, purple, or new potatoes would work as well (you just want the rounds to be large enough to hold the toppings). Fingerling potatoes can work if you cut them lengthwise.

Instead of spinach, use organic kale.

In place of black olives, use green or kalamata olives.

Substitute chives or parsley for cilantro.

Instead of red onions, use yellow or white onions.

Instead of Cilantro Cream, add your favorite store-bought plant-based cheese or plant-based sour cream, or some homemade cashew cheese (see the recipe for Plant-tastic Mushroom Ziti Bake on page 150).

Prep Ahead

Cut the potatoes the day before and store them in the refrigerator in an airtight container for up to 24 hours.

If using the Cilantro Cream, make it ahead of time and store it in the refrigerator for 5 to 7 days.

Double the Batch

If you want to make more, then double all of the ingredients, but note that when starting with the raw potato rounds, you'll have to use two parchment-lined baking sheets to bake them the first time around. They shrink upon baking; therefore, you'll be able to transfer all of the baked potato rounds to one baking sheet before adding the toppings.

Storage

These nachos are best when enjoyed immediately after baking. If you have leftovers, store them in an airtight container in the refrigerator for up to 3 days and reheat them at 400°F for 10 to 15 minutes.

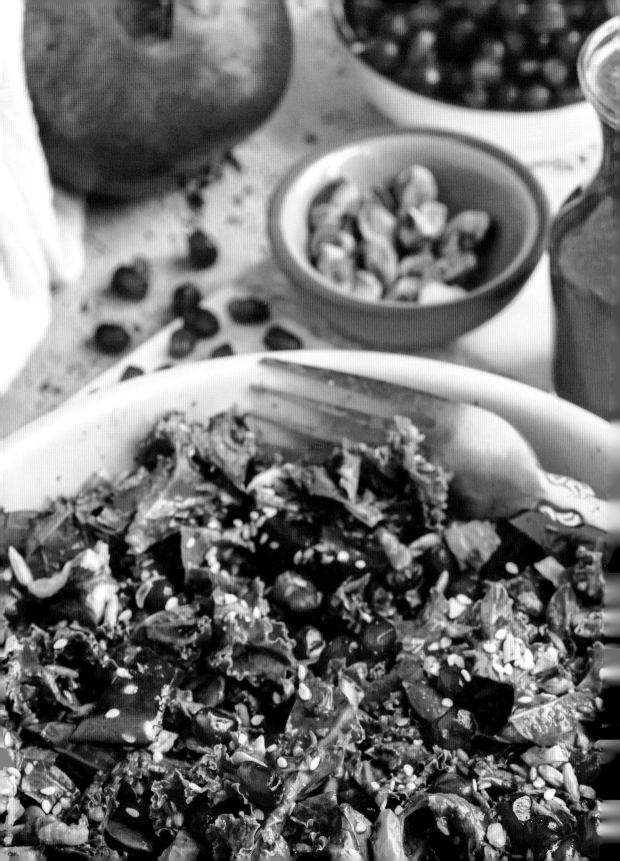

SATISFYING SALADS

FILL ME WITH WARMTH TEMPEH AND KALE SALAD

Warming and *comforting* are not usually synonymous with *salad*, but it's good to break the rules every now and then when it comes to delicious, plant-based cooking. This warm salad offers tons of flavor, a variety of textures, and plenty of nutritional benefits with tempeh, kale, radish, and red onion. It's refreshing and hearty at the same time, making it a versatile salad that's great for any season, whether it's a warm summer evening or a chilly winter night. Add your favorite whole grain like organic quinoa or wheat berries to make it a complete meal!

Serves 2 **Prep time** 15 minutes **Cooking time** 10 minutes

8 ounces organic tempeh, cut in half lengthwise then halved again through the middle.

Marinade

1 tablespoon organic mellow white or chickpea miso

2 tablespoons organic reduced-sodium tamari or coconut aminos

2 tablespoons organic rice vinegar

1 tablespoon freshly squeezed lime juice

1 tablespoon maple syrup

1 tablespoon gochujang, sriracha, or chili paste, optional

¼ teaspoon garlic powder

¼ teaspoon ground ginger

Salad Ingredients

4 cups kale, stemmed and finely chopped

1 teaspoon extra virgin olive oil, optional

½ lime, juiced

2 pinches of salt, optional

½ cup radish, thinly sliced

¼ cup red onion, diced

2 tablespoons sesame seeds

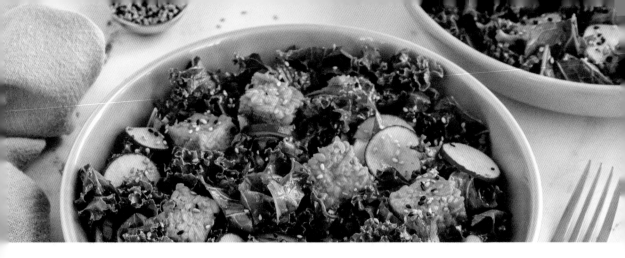

1. Boil or steam the tempeh: Submerge the tempeh in enough water to cover them or place in a steamer basket in a pot with water. Cook for 10 minutes.
2. In the meantime, whisk all of the marinade ingredients in a medium bowl with 2 tablespoons of water until all of the miso has dissolved.
3. Once the tempeh is finished cooking, remove, drain, and transfer to a cutting board. Cut into 1-inch cubes.
4. Transfer the tempeh to a shallow dish and pour ¾ of the marinade over top. Stir to coat the tempeh. Let sit for 20 minutes.
5. Meanwhile, in a large bowl, drizzle the kale with the oil and lime juice, and sprinkle 2 pinches of salt on top, if desired. Massage until the kale is tender, about 30 seconds.
6. Add the radish and red onion. Toss.
7. In a large skillet over medium heat, heat the tempeh, stirring occasionally, until just warm, about 1 to 2 minutes. (Keep the heat on medium or medium-low to prevent the tempeh from sticking. Depending on your pan, you may need to lightly coat it with oil, but make sure to wipe off any excess oil with a paper towel.)
8. Toss the tempeh with the kale salad. Drizzle the remaining marinade over the salad and sprinkle with sesame seeds.

CHEF'S NOTES

Substitutions

Use another leafy green in place of kale, such as spinach, chard, or mixed greens.

Use shallots in place of onion.

If You Like It Saucy

Double the marinade recipe, pour half over the tempeh, and reserve the other half for the salad. (This salad is pretty light on the dressing, but just enough in our opinion.)

Whole-Food Sweetener

Use date paste in place of maple syrup.

Prep Ahead

Prepare the tempeh the day before and let it marinate in the refrigerator overnight for even more flavor.

Storage

Store leftovers in an airtight container in the refrigerator for up to 5 days.

UNCOMPLICATED CRUNCHY KALE SLAW

Carrots, kale, and cabbage (talk about alliteration!) make this Uncomplicated Crunchy Kale Slaw spectacular. The inclusion of nutty hemp seeds and sesame seeds adds more crunch and healthy fats that help to bring out the flavors in this dish. One of the (many) reasons we love this recipe so much is that it requires no cooking, just a little shredding, making this dish one that provides tons of nutrition in exchange for minimal preparation. Enjoy it solo, as a side dish, or on top of tacos and wraps.

Serves 4 **Prep time** 15 minutes **Cooking time** none

3 cups kale, stemmed and shredded

2 teaspoons freshly squeezed lemon or lime juice

1 cup red cabbage, shredded

1 cup carrots, shredded

¼ cup hemp seeds

¼ cup sunflower seeds

Dressing

1½ tablespoons tahini

1½ teaspoons Dijon mustard

1½ tablespoons organic apple cider vinegar

1 tablespoon maple syrup

1 teaspoon ground turmeric

1. Add the kale to a large bowl. Squeeze the lemon or lime juice over top and massage the kale until the leaves are tender, about 30 to 60 seconds.
2. Add the cabbage and carrots and toss.
3. Make the dressing: Add all ingredients to a small bowl with 1 to 2 tablespoons of water and whisk until smooth.
4. Pour the dressing over the kale, cabbage, and carrot mixture. Toss thoroughly to combine.
5. Add the hemp seeds and sunflower seeds and toss once more.
6. Serve as a side slaw or as a topping for tacos or veggie burgers.

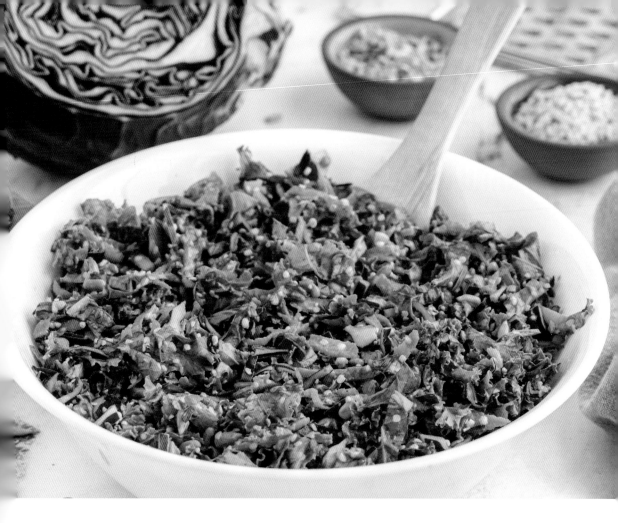

CHEF'S NOTES

Substitutions

Instead of kale, use another leafy green of choice.

Use green cabbage in place of red cabbage.

Substitute pumpkin seeds for sunflower seeds.

Use brown mustard in place of Dijon mustard.

Whole-Food Sweetener

Use date paste in place of maple syrup.

Prep Ahead

Make the dressing ahead of time and store it in an airtight container in the refrigerator for up to 5 days.

Shred the slaw ingredients ahead of time and store them in an airtight container in the refrigerator for up to 2 days.

Storage

Store leftovers in an airtight container in the refrigerator for up to 3 days.

LEMONY BASIL FARRO SALAD

Looking for new salad inspiration? Chewy and nutty farro is the hearty base for this deliciously simple salad, tossed together with white beans, spicy arugula, sweet tomatoes, savory basil, and bright lemon. These diverse ingredients come together to create a salad that is as lively as it is unique! Enjoy this dish by itself, alongside your main course, or as an afternoon pick-me-up.

Serves 4 **Prep time** 20 minutes **Cooking time** none

Salad

3 cups cooked farro

1½ cups grape tomatoes, halved

1 medium cucumber, peeled if waxed and cut into ¼-inch pieces

1½ cups home-cooked or canned white beans, drained and rinsed

1 cup green onion, chopped (use the green and white parts)

2 cups arugula

Dressing

½ cup fresh basil, chopped

¼ cup tahini

2 garlic cloves

½ cup freshly squeezed lemon juice

½ cup walnut pieces

1 tablespoon maple syrup

¼ teaspoon salt, optional

¼ teaspoon ground black pepper, optional

1. In a large bowl, add all the salad ingredients—farro, tomatoes, cucumber, white beans, green onion, and arugula. Toss to combine.

2. In a food processor or blender, add all the dressing ingredients and blend until smooth. Taste and boost flavors of your choice (extra lemon, basil, salt, or pepper).

3. Pour the dressing on top of the farro salad bowl and mix well.

4. Divide between serving bowls and enjoy!

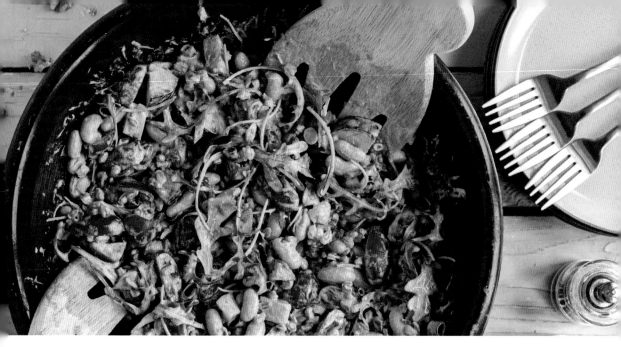

CHEF'S NOTES

Substitutions

Instead of farro, use organic wheat berries, quinoa, Kamut, or another grain.

In place of arugula, use spinach, kale, or red leaf lettuce. Or a combination!

In place of tomato or cucumber, use whatever delicious vegetables you have on hand, such as radish, asparagus, broccoli, or red cabbage.

Layer It Up

Add sliced avocado for some creaminess to complement the cucumber crunch.

Add more herbs, such as cilantro, parsley, or dill.

Stir in some kimchi for a little spice and probiotics.

Top with red pepper flakes for some spice.

Stir in your favorite nuts or seeds like pistachios or pumpkin seeds.

Prep Ahead

Make the farro ahead of time and store it in an airtight container in the refrigerator for up to 3 days or freeze for up to 3 months.

If using homemade beans, make them ahead of time and store in an airtight container in the refrigerator for up to 3 days before making this recipe or freeze for up to 3 months.

Make the dressing ahead of time and store it in an airtight container in the refrigerator for up to 3 days before making this recipe.

Whole-Food Sweetener

Use date paste in place of maple syrup.

Storage

Store leftovers in an airtight container in the refrigerator for up to 3 days.

HEARTY WILD RICE, MUSHROOM, AND BABY BROCCOLI SALAD

Superfood salads can be made with nearly any plant-based ingredients because, in our humble opinion, all fruits and vegetables are super thanks to their ability to heal and nourish. This salad is no exception! There is no lettuce in sight, but this hearty dish offers all the bright, crunchy, creamy, and colorful elements of a traditional salad. It's filling, nourishing, and has plenty of flavor to make your belly happy, make your taste buds sing, and make your body dance.

Serves 4 **Prep time** 20 minutes **Cooking time** 45 minutes

Dressing

2 tablespoons tahini
¼ cup apple cider vinegar
2 teaspoons Dijon mustard
1 tablespoon maple syrup
¼ teaspoon onion powder

Rice

1 cup rinsed wild rice
3 cups unsalted or low-sodium
   vegetable broth

Veggies

1 bunch baby broccoli, stems cut into
   ¼-inch pieces and florets cuts into 1-inch
   pieces (separate stems from the florets)
1 cup carrots, thinly sliced
1 cup mushrooms, sliced
1 tablespoon reduced-sodium tamari or
   coconut aminos

Toppings

4 tablespoons hemp seeds
2 to 4 tablespoons freshly chopped
   herbs of choice (parsley, cilantro, basil),
   optional

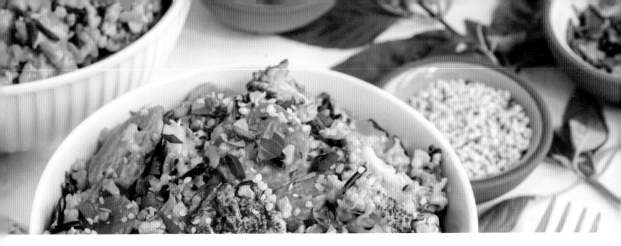

1. Whisk all dressing ingredients in a small bowl with 1 to 2 tablespoons of water until the tahini is dissolved. Set aside.

2. In a medium pan, bring the rice and vegetable broth to a boil then simmer, cover, and cook on medium heat for about 45 minutes or until the liquid is absorbed. Set aside to cool.

3. Meanwhile, in a large pan on medium heat, cook the broccoli stems, carrots, and mushrooms for 3 minutes, stirring often. Add 1 to 2 tablespoons of water as needed to deglaze the pan.

4. Add the tamari, broccoli florets, and 1 cup of water. Partially cover and let steam for 10 minutes or until the carrots are tender.

5. Remove the vegetables from the heat. Drain any excess liquid. Transfer the rice and vegetables to a large bowl.

6. Pour the dressing over top and stir well. Sprinkle with hemp seeds and chopped herbs of your choice.

CHEF'S NOTES

Substitutions

Substitute brown or black rice or another whole grain in place of wild rice.

Use regular broccoli in place of baby broccoli.

For the mushrooms, use cremini, button, or portobello.

Substitute red or yellow pepper for the carrots.

Consistency

You may need to add one tablespoon of water or more, depending on your preferred consistency.

Whole-Food Sweetener

Use date paste in place of maple syrup.

Prep Ahead

Make the rice ahead of time and store in an airtight container in the refrigerator for up to 3 days or freeze for up to 3 months.

Make the dressing ahead of time and store it in an airtight container in the refrigerator for up to 5 days.

Storage

Store leftovers in an airtight container in the refrigerator for up to 5 days or freeze them for up to 1 month.

MINTY FRESH STRAWBERRY SALAD

Discovering new flavor combinations can be one of many ways to keep plant-based eating exciting, vibrant, and intriguing. Combining sweet strawberries with refreshing mint and drizzling savory, nutty, citrus dressing on top creates a new spin on traditional salads. Strawberries and mint are a juicy and cooling flavor combination that is perfect for a light meal. Enjoy this salad with a mild-flavored bean, on top of hearty whole grains, or on a bed of delicate mixed greens.

Serves 4 **Prep time** 10 minutes **Cooking time** none

2 cups strawberries, hulled and quartered

¼ cup red onion, diced

2 tablespoons fresh mint leaves, minced

2 tablespoons fresh basil, minced, optional

1 sprinkle of salt, optional

Dressing

1 tablespoon tahini

2 tablespoons maple syrup

1 tablespoon freshly squeezed lime juice

Topping

2 tablespoons slivered or sliced almonds

1. Combine the strawberries, onion, mint, and basil in a medium bowl. Add a sprinkle of salt, if desired.

2. In a small bowl, whisk together the tahini, maple syrup, and lime juice until well combined.

3. Divide the berry mixture between two bowls and drizzle with the dressing. Top with slivered or sliced almonds.

CHEF'S NOTES

Substitutions

Instead of red onion, use shallots or yellow onion.

Instead of basil, use cilantro.

Sprinkle sunflower seeds or chopped walnuts over top instead of almonds.

Use lemon juice in place of lime juice.

Prep Ahead

Prepare the tahini dressing ahead of time, cover, and store it in the refrigerator for up to 5 days.

Whole-Food Sweetener

Use date paste in place of maple syrup.

Storage

Store leftovers in an airtight container in the refrigerator for up to 2 days.

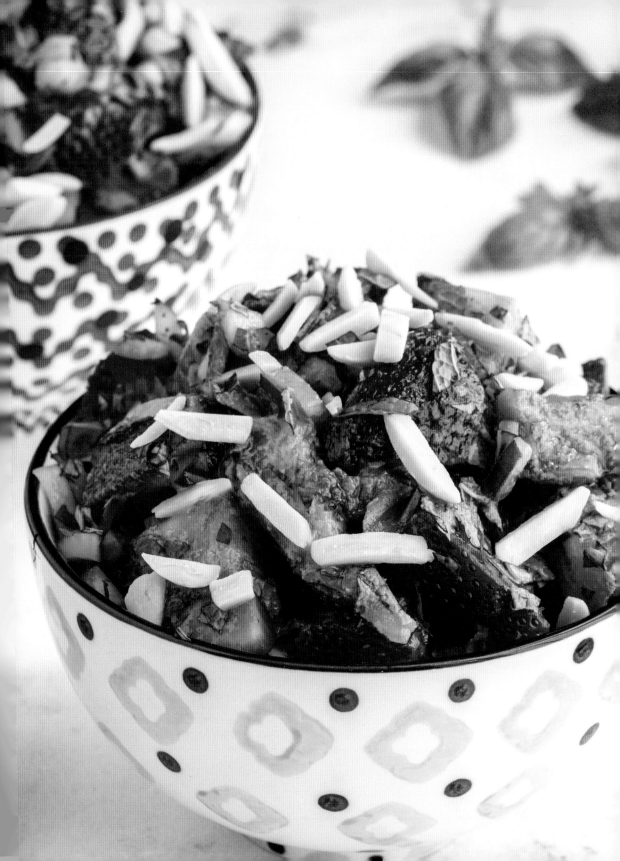

FEELING UPBEET AND LIVELY LENTIL SALAD

If you're not a fan of beets, that might change after trying this dish. Roasting them brings out natural sweetness that shines through with the Lemon Shallot Vinaigrette. The dressing has a touch of natural sweetness from the dates, but if you'd like a bit more, consider adding fruit-juice-sweetened dried cranberries, apricots, or figs. This hearty and comforting salad has no shortage of superfood nutrition and makes a supremely comforting plant-based meal or side dish.

Serves 2 **Prep time** 20 minutes **Cooking time** 60 minutes

Beets

4 small beets, scrubbed and tops removed

¼ cup unsalted or low-sodium vegetable broth

1 lemon, juiced

3 to 4 sprigs fresh thyme

½ large red onion, sliced

Lemon Shallot Vinaigrette

1 garlic clove

¼ cup shallots, chopped

¼ cup freshly squeezed lemon juice

1 tablespoon balsamic vinegar

1 tablespoon sherry or red wine vinegar

¼ cup date paste

2 tablespoons tahini

¼ teaspoon salt, optional

¼ teaspoon ground black pepper, optional

Salad

4 cups mixed greens or lettuce of your choice

1 cup home-cooked or BPA-free canned lentils, drained and rinsed

¼ cup raw walnuts

1. Preheat the oven to 325°F.

2. Tear off a large enough piece of foil to make a "boat" to steam-roast the beets. Lay the same size piece of parchment paper on top of the foil. Place the beets inside the foil/parchment paper. Add the vegetable broth, lemon juice, thyme, and a pinch of salt. Wrap the beets so there is room for steam to rise within the tin foil and tighten the edges.

3. Place the beet boat on a large parchment-lined baking sheet. Spread out red onion slices on the sheet next to the beets (they should stay outside of the foil so they get crispy). Roast for 45 to 60 minutes (depending on the size of the beets). Check the onions halfway through and move them around if the onions around the outer edges of the baking sheet are browning and getting crispier than the onions toward the center of the sheet. When the beets are fork tender, remove from the oven and set aside to cool in the foil package.

4. In the meantime, blend all the dressing ingredients in a food processor or blender until smooth. Taste and adjust the ingredients to your liking (more lemon for acid, more date paste for sweetness, or more tahini for creaminess).

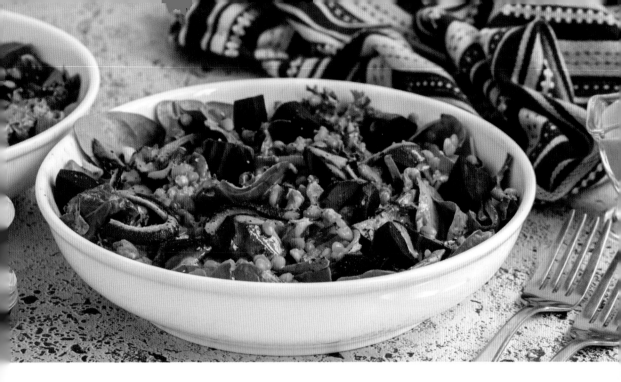

5. Once the beets have cooled, if desired, carefully remove the skins, then cut the beets into quarters or slices.

6. Split all ingredients between two plates or bowls. Add the desired amount of salad dressing and pepper over the top.

CHEF'S NOTES

Substitutions

Instead of lentils, use your favorite legume or one that you have on hand.

Instead of mixed greens, try butter lettuce, romaine, or organic kale.

Instead of thyme, use rosemary or oregano.

Use 3 tablespoons of maple syrup in place of date paste.

In place of walnuts, try chopped pistachios, almonds, pecans, or hazelnuts.

Onion Options

Steam the onions: If desired, you can steam the onions with the beets. You'll just need a little extra foil and parchment to ensure you can close the foil over both the onions and beets. The onions will turn purple from the beets and take on some beet flavor. They'll also have a soft texture as opposed to the crunchy texture from dry roasting.

Use raw onions instead of roasted or steamed ones (this is also delicious and good for those of you who love raw onion flavor).

Prep Ahead

Make the beets ahead of time and store them in the refrigerator for 7 to 10 days.

Make the dressing ahead of time and store it in the refrigerator for 7 to 10 days.

Storage

Store leftovers in an airtight container in the refrigerator for up to 3 days.

SUPER SEED AUTUMN SALAD WITH TART POMEGRANATE DRESSING

Maybe we should rename this dish "Antioxidant-Powered Kale Salad" since just about every ingredient in this dish is powered with antioxidants. This simple and delicious dish is bursting with sweet, nutty, and earthy flavors. It offers crunchy, creamy, and silky textures, and provides plenty of iron, folate, and vitamin C. What's more, it only takes 15 minutes to create. The power of plants is real, folks!

Serves 2 **Prep time** 15 minutes **Cooking time** none

Pomegranate Vinaigrette

2 tablespoons tahini

¼ cup freshly squeezed or unsweetened bottled pomegranate juice

2 tablespoons balsamic vinegar

1 tablespoon maple syrup

½ teaspoon garlic powder

¼ teaspoon onion powder

¼ teaspoon dried oregano

Salt to taste, optional

Ground black pepper to taste, optional

Salad Ingredients

4 cups kale, stemmed and chopped

½ cup beets, cooked and sliced

2 tablespoons pomegranate seeds

1 tablespoon raw or toasted sunflower seeds

1 tablespoon raw or toasted pumpkin seeds

1 tablespoon raw or toasted sesame seeds

2 tablespoons chopped raw or toasted walnuts

2 tablespoons shelled raw or toasted pistachios

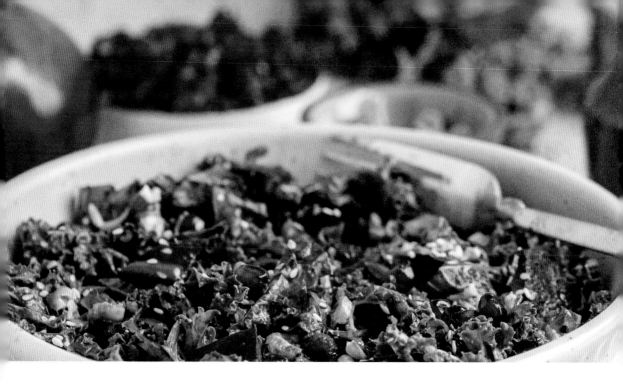

1. Add the vinaigrette ingredients to a 16-ounce mason jar or a medium bowl. Put the lid on the mason jar and shake it or whisk the ingredients in the bowl until all of the tahini is dissolved.

2. Add the kale and 1 tablespoon of the dressing to a large bowl. Massage the dressing into the kale for 30 to 60 seconds until the leaves soften.

3. Add the remaining salad ingredients (beets, pomegranate seeds, sunflower seeds, pumpkin seeds, sesame seeds, walnuts, and pistachios). Mix well.

4. Divide the salad between two medium bowls.

5. Pour the desired amount of dressing on top of each salad.

CHEF'S NOTES

Toasting the Nuts and Seeds

Most nuts and larger seeds should be toasted in a pan on medium heat for 3 to 5 minutes or until fragrant.

To toast sesame seeds, use a small pan and medium-low heat. Toast for 2 to 3 minutes or until fragrant.

Whole-Food Sweetener

Use date paste in place of maple syrup.

Add More Nutrition

Add shredded carrots to the salad.

Add baked squash.

Top with flax or hemp seeds.

Storage

Store leftovers in an airtight container in the refrigerator for up to 3 days.

Extra dressing should be kept in its own container in the refrigerator for 5 to 7 days.

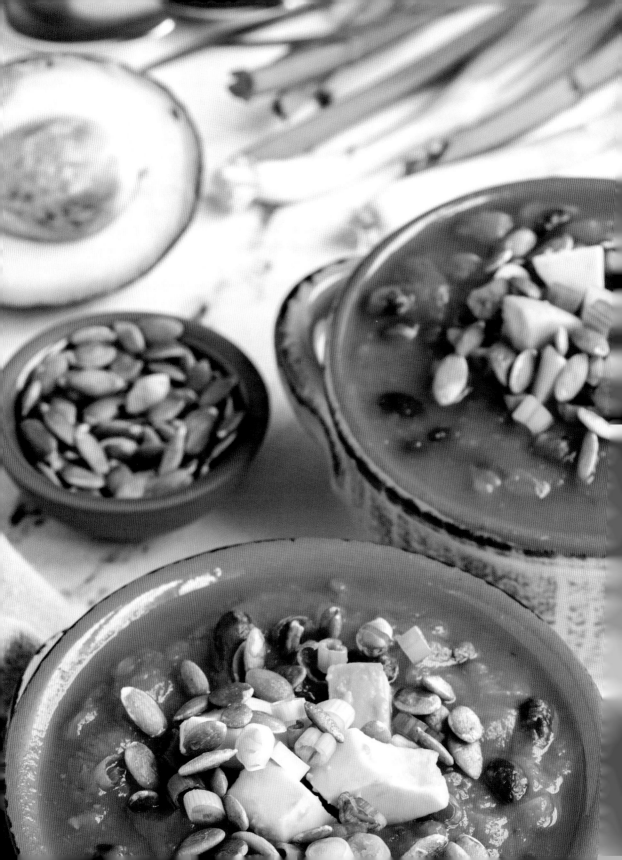

SAVORY SOUPS
AND STEWS

PERFECTLY SPICED SPINACH LENTIL SOUP

What's not to love about soup? It's often easy to prepare, bursting with flavor, and warm and comforting. It's also a simple and tasty way to include a wide variety of nutrient-dense, plant-based ingredients. This soup checks all those boxes—a flavorful and rich one-pot, nutrient-packed dish that can soothe body and soul. Enjoy it with a warm and crusty piece of whole grain bread for an extra special soup experience.

Serves 4 **Prep time** 10 minutes **Cooking time** 70 minutes

1 teaspoon mustard seeds

1 teaspoon cumin seeds

1 teaspoon fennel seeds

1 chopped medium white or yellow onion

3 carrots, chopped

2 stalks celery, chopped

3 garlic cloves, minced

1 teaspoon dried oregano

¼ teaspoon ground cayenne pepper or crushed red pepper flakes, optional

1 28-ounce can crushed tomatoes

2 cups unsalted or low-sodium vegetable broth

2 cups dry green or brown lentils

2 cups spinach, chopped

Salt to taste, optional

Ground black pepper to taste, optional

Crushed red pepper to taste, optional

Toppings

Nutritional yeast to taste, optional

Freshly chopped basil to taste, optional

1. In a large pot over medium-high heat, toast the mustard, cumin, and fennel seeds for one minute, tossing a few times to evenly toast.
2. Add the onion, carrots, and celery, and cook them until the onion is soft and tender, about 5 minutes.
3. Stir in the garlic, oregano, and cayenne or red pepper flakes and cook for another 30 seconds.
4. Stir in the tomatoes, broth, lentils, and 4 cups of water. Bring to a boil, then reduce the heat and let simmer, uncovered, for 1 hour.
5. Remove the pot from the heat and stir in the spinach. When the spinach is tender, the soup is ready for serving.
6. Add salt, pepper, and red pepper flakes to taste. Top with nutritional yeast and fresh basil.

CHEF'S NOTES

Substitutions

Substitute mung beans for lentils.

Use kale in place of spinach.

Storage

Store leftovers in an airtight container in the refrigerator for up to 5 days or freeze them for up to 3 months.

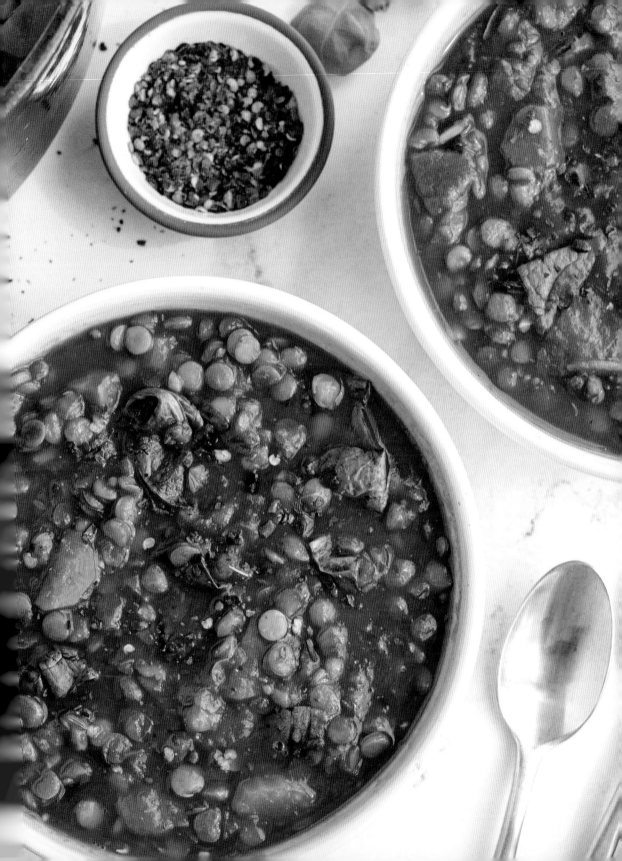

BUTTER BEAN ME UP ONE-POT SOUP

Buttery and rich, yet refreshing and light, Butter Bean Me Up One-Pot Soup brings together delectable flavors and textures to create a soup that might become a staple in your family's meal rotation. It's also super filling and satisfying given the plentiful fiber and protein content from those hearty butter beans!

Serves 4 **Prep time** 15 minutes **Cooking time** 20 minutes

1½ cups yellow onion, chopped

1 cup carrots, diced

1 bunch Swiss chard, stemmed and chopped (separate leaves from stems and reserve both parts)

1 tablespoon garlic, minced

1½ tablespoons fresh thyme, minced

5 cups unsalted or low-sodium vegetable broth

3 cups home-cooked or canned butter beans, drained and rinsed

1 teaspoon ground turmeric

½ teaspoon crushed red pepper flakes, optional

¼ teaspoon salt, optional

¼ teaspoon ground black pepper, optional

1 tablespoon freshly squeezed lemon juice

⅓ cup hulled hemp seeds

1. Heat the onion, carrots, and Swiss chard stems in a large pot on medium-high until the onions are translucent, about 4 to 5 minutes.

2. Stir in the garlic and thyme. Cook for 1 minute.

3. Add the vegetable broth, butter beans, turmeric, and optional red pepper flakes, salt, and pepper.

Bring the soup to a boil, then lower the heat and let it simmer, uncovered, for 10 to 15 minutes.

4. Remove the pot from the heat and stir in the Swiss chard leaves, lemon juice, and hemp seeds.

5. Taste and boost your seasonings of choice.

CHEF'S NOTES

Substitutions

Instead of Swiss chard, try kale, mustard, or collard greens.

Substitute white onion or shallots for the yellow onion.

Instead of butter beans, use great northern, navy, or cannellini beans.

Prep Ahead

Chop the onions and Swiss chard (separate stems and leaves) ahead of time and store them in an airtight container in the refrigerator for up to 48 hours before making the recipe.

Storage

Store leftovers in an airtight container in the refrigerator for up to 5 days or freeze them for up to 30 days.

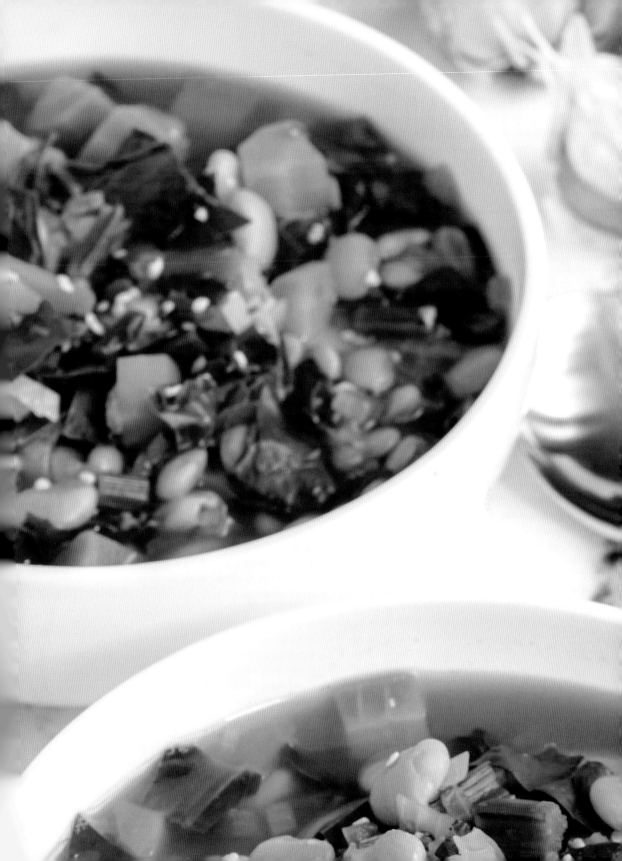

SWEET AND SAVORY PEANUT SOUP

Who knew that naturally sweet and nutty peanut butter could pair so well with savory tomatoes to create the most exquisite culinary experience? This soup was inspired by a staple food from West Africa, where it's called *domodah* or *tigadegena* meaning "peanut butter sauce" (*tige* is "peanut," *dege* is "paste," and *na* is "sauce"). It can be made with or without meat, but it always includes peanuts and tomatoes. It's delicious hot or cold, as a main meal or appetizer, or for breakfast or dinner. Yes, a few members of the Food Revolution Network team have enjoyed cold leftovers for breakfast and claim it's just as good, if not better, the next day.

Serves 4 **Prep time** 15 minutes **Cooking time** 40 minutes

Sautéed Vegetables

¼ cup unsalted or low-sodium vegetable broth

1 yellow onion, chopped

4 garlic cloves, minced

2 tablespoons fresh ginger, minced

1 teaspoon ground turmeric

¼ teaspoon salt, optional

¼ teaspoon ground black pepper, optional

½ teaspoon crushed red pepper flakes, optional

Soup

4 cups unsalted, vegetable broth

2 medium sweet potatoes, cubed

6 ounces tomato paste

¾ cup smooth or crunchy unsweetened peanut butter

1½ cups home-cooked or canned chickpeas, drained and rinsed

1 teaspoon sweet paprika

1 teaspoon ground cumin

½ teaspoon salt, optional

3 cups spinach, chopped

Garnish

½ cup fresh cilantro, chopped

½ cup green onion, chopped

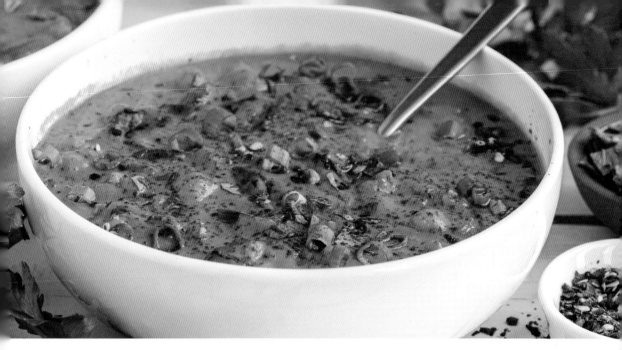

1. In a large pot on medium-high heat, add the onion and ¼ cup vegetable broth. Turn down the heat to medium, and cook 1 to 2 minutes until the onion is translucent.

2. Stir in the garlic, ginger, turmeric, and salt, pepper, and red pepper flakes so they coat the onions and garlic. Cook 2 to 3 minutes on medium-low.

3. Add 4 cups of vegetable broth and 2 cups of water; bring to a boil. Add the cubed sweet potato and cook until the potatoes are soft, about 10 minutes.

4. Meanwhile, mix the tomato paste and peanut butter together in a small bowl until well combined.

5. Add the peanut butter and tomato paste mixture to the soup and stir until they're completely dissolved.

6. Stir in the chickpeas, paprika, cumin, and salt. Simmer on low for 15 minutes; the soup will thicken.

7. Stir in the spinach, one cup at a time, and cook until the spinach is tender.

8. Top with cilantro and green onion, as well as another dash of paprika and red pepper flakes for more spice.

CHEF'S NOTES

Substitutions

In place of chickpeas, try lentils or baked tofu pieces.

Instead of spinach, use kale.

In place of sweet potato, use butternut squash or purple potatoes.

Layer It Up

Top with chopped peanuts, almonds, pecans, or sesame seeds.

Spoon the soup into a baked squash boat.

Storage

Store leftovers in an airtight container in the refrigerator for up to 7 days or in the freezer for up to 30 days.

SUPERGREEN MUSHROOM AND POTATO SOUP

Don't let it fool you—this soup may have minimal ingredients and require little cooking, but it's powered with nutrition, flavors, and textures. With the leafy greens, mushrooms, garlic, onions, and herbs, it's one to keep in your library for when you need serious nourishment with minimal time investment.

Serves 4 **Prep time** 20 minutes **Cooking time** 20 minutes

1 cup celery, chopped

1 cup yellow or white onion, chopped

1 bunch Swiss chard, stemmed and chopped (separate leaves from stems and reserve both parts)

4 garlic cloves, minced

3 cups broccoli, cut into 1-inch florets

2 cups cremini, button, or portobello mushrooms, chopped

1 tablespoon vegan Worcestershire sauce

1 teaspoon onion powder

1 tablespoon fresh thyme, minced

8 cups unsalted or low-sodium vegetable broth

2 cups red potatoes, cut into 1-inch cubes

1. Heat the celery, onion, and Swiss chard stems in a large stockpot on medium-high heat, stirring frequently until the onions are translucent, about 3 to 5 minutes. Add 1 to 2 tablespoons of water as needed to deglaze the pot.

2. Stir in the garlic, turn down the heat to medium, and cook for 1 minute.

3. Stir in the broccoli, mushrooms, Worcestershire sauce, onion powder, and thyme, and cook for 1 minute.

4. Pour in the vegetable broth and turn up the heat to high. Once the broth is boiling, add the potatoes and lower the heat to a simmer until the potatoes are tender, about 10 minutes.

5. Stir in the Swiss chard leaves, cooking until tender.

6. Taste the soup and boost it with additional seasoning or some salt and pepper, if you like.

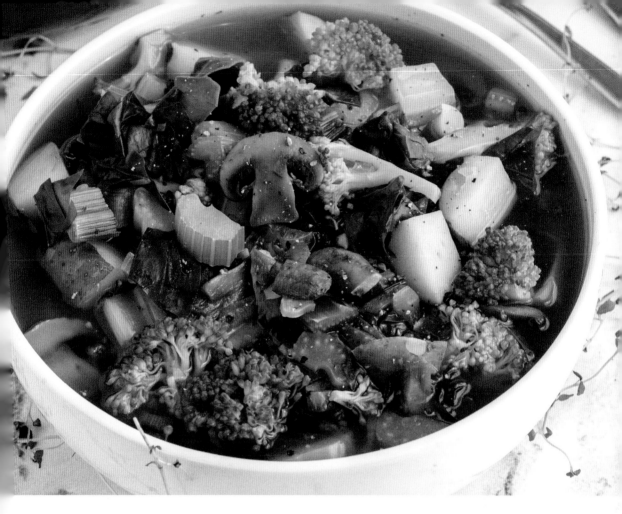

CHEF'S NOTES

Substitutions

In place of red potatoes, use any potato variety you enjoy.

In place of potatoes, add your favorite (cooked) whole grain, like barley, brown rice, or farro.

Use kale, mustard, or collard greens in place of Swiss chard.

Substitute cauliflower for broccoli.

Use fresh rosemary or oregano in place of thyme.

Prep Ahead

Chop your celery, onion, Swiss chard (separate the leaves and stems), broccoli, and mushrooms ahead of time and store in airtight containers in the refrigerator for up to 2 days.

Storage

Store leftovers in an airtight container in the refrigerator for up to 5 days.

CREAMY DREAMY ARUGULA AND WHITE BEAN SOUP

Plant-based foods are pretty magical in the way that they can create the creamiest textures without the need for any cream, and Creamy Dreamy Arugula and White Bean Soup is a prime example. Potatoes, white beans, and hemp seeds lend to the creamy texture while celery, arugula, and cilantro contribute their pretty green hues. All of the ingredients offer even more than magical textures and colors, and that's their bountiful nutrition!

Serves 4 **Prep time** 15 minutes **Cooking time** 20 minutes

1 cup yellow or white onion, chopped

1 cup celery, sliced

3 garlic cloves, roughly minced

¼ teaspoon celery seed, optional

1½ cups red, Yukon Gold, or russet potatoes, cubed

1½ cups home-cooked or canned white beans, drained and rinsed

4 cups unsalted or low-sodium vegetable broth

3 cups arugula, roughly chopped

½ cup fresh cilantro, roughly chopped, optional

Salt to taste, optional

Ground black pepper to taste, optional

¼ cup avocado, cut into ½-inch cubes

¼ cup tomatoes, diced

2 tablespoons hulled hemp seeds

4 lemon wedges

1. Heat a large pot on medium-high heat. Add the onion and celery, cooking for 5 to 7 minutes or until the celery is tender.

2. Add the garlic and optional celery seed and cook for 1 minute.

3. Add the potatoes, beans, and vegetable broth. Bring the soup to a boil, then reduce the heat to simmer. Cook until the potatoes are tender, about 10 minutes.

4. Add the arugula and optional cilantro, and simmer for an additional 2 minutes or until the arugula is bright green.

5. Let the soup cool a bit before transferring it to a blender. Blend until smooth and creamy. Taste and add salt and pepper, if using.

6. Divide the soup between four bowls and top it with avocado, tomato, and a sprinkle of hemp seeds.

7. Serve with lemon wedges.

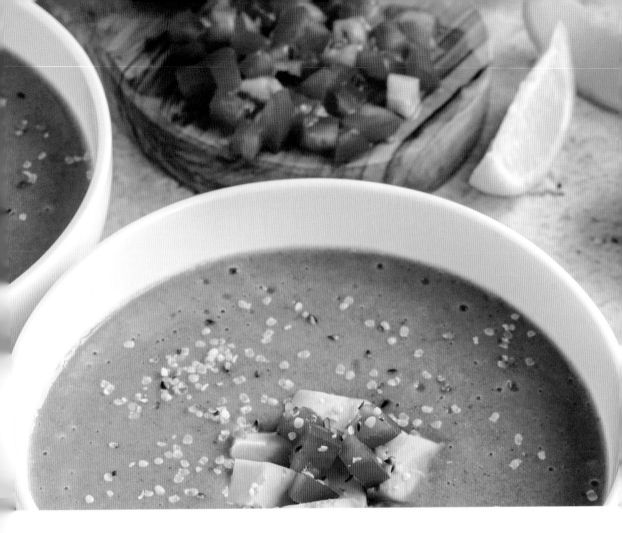

CHEF'S NOTES

Substitutions

For the onion, use yellow, white, or red onion. Or use shallots in place of onion.

Instead of arugula, try spinach or kale.

In place of white beans, use great northern, navy, or cannellini beans.

Substitute parsley or basil for cilantro.

For the tomatoes, use diced Roma, cherry, garden, or any variety you have on hand.

Prep Ahead

Prepare your beans and vegetable broth ahead of time if you're planning to use homemade versions.

Storage

Store leftovers in an airtight container in the refrigerator for up to 3 days or freeze them for up to 1 month.

SUNSET GLOW ROOT VEGGIE SOUP WITH TOASTED SUNFLOWER SEEDS

Warm your heart and your belly with this comforting, jewel-toned, creamy soup that is fiber filled and phytonutrient rich thanks to sweet potatoes and carrots. Adding a pinch of vibrant microgreens just before serving adds another pop of color plus a generous amount of nutrition. Sprinkling sunflower seeds on top adds even more nutrition plus a fun crunch and nutty flavor.

Serves 4 **Prep time** 20 minutes **Cooking time** 25 minutes

2 pounds sweet potatoes, cut into 1-inch cubes

2 large carrots, sliced

Salt to taste, optional

Ground black pepper to taste, optional

1 teaspoon mustard seeds

1 large yellow onion, thinly sliced

4 medium garlic cloves, minced

1 teaspoon ground turmeric

1 teaspoon ground cumin

5 cups unsalted or low-sodium vegetable broth

2 tablespoons raw sunflower seeds

¼ cup microgreens (see Chef's Notes)

1. Preheat the oven to 425°F. Evenly spread out sweet potatoes and carrots on a parchment-lined baking sheet. Sprinkle lightly with salt and pepper, if desired. Roast until tender, about 25 minutes.

2. Meanwhile, heat a large saucepan over medium-high heat. Add the mustard seeds and cook until fragrant, about 1 minute.

3. Add the onion and cook until translucent, about 3 to 5 minutes. Stir in the garlic, turmeric, and cumin and cook for 1 minute.

4. Add the vegetable broth and simmer for 5 minutes. Turn off the heat and set aside.

5. Heat a small pan over medium heat. Add the sunflower seeds and toast them, tossing occasionally, for 1 to 2 minutes until they're golden brown. Remove the pan from the heat and set aside.

6. Once the roasted sweet potatoes and carrots are finished cooking, transfer them to the saucepan with the onions and garlic. Bring the sweet potato, carrot, and onion mixture to a boil, then turn down the heat to simmer for 5 minutes.

7. Transfer the soup to a blender and blend until very smooth. You may need to do this in 2 to 3 batches. If needed, add more vegetable broth to reach the consistency you desire. Alternatively, use an immersion blender to keep everything in one place.

8. Ladle the soup into bowls and garnish with the toasted sunflower seeds. Scatter some microgreens on each bowl.

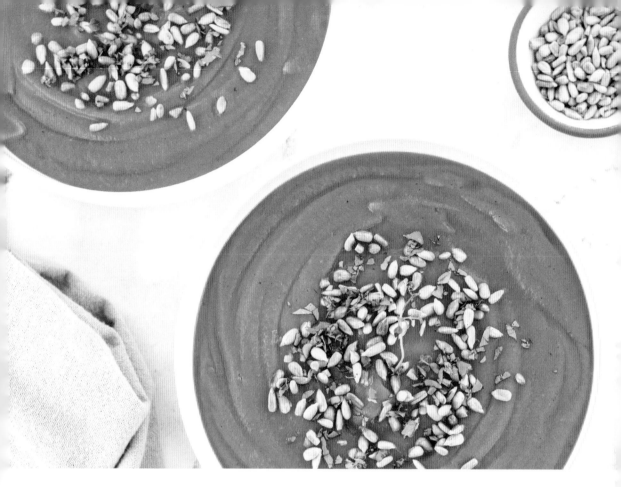

CHEF'S NOTES

Substitutions

Use butternut squash in place of the sweet potato and/or carrots. If using butternut squash sauce in place of sweet potato, use only 4 cups of vegetable broth, reserving the last cup only if needed during the blending process if you'd like a thinner consistency.

Instead of yellow onion, use shallots or white onion (about 1½ cups).

Microgreens

Use arugula, radish, basil, sunflower, broccoli, alfalfa, or any microgreen of your choice.

Prep Ahead

Roast the sweet potatoes and carrots ahead of time and store in an airtight container in the refrigerator for up to 48 hours.

Toast the sunflower seeds and store in an airtight container in the refrigerator for up to 2 weeks.

Storage

Store leftovers in an airtight container in the refrigerator for up to 5 days or freeze them for up to 30 days.

GOURD-GEOUS NOURISHING PUMPKIN CHILI

If you're a chili lover, you probably appreciate lots of (plant-based) variations because they're all wholesome, nourishing, delicious, and satisfying. Gourd-geous Nourishing Pumpkin Chili is all that plus it goes the extra mile by including nutrient-rich pumpkin. This chili is overflowing with carotenoids from the pumpkin and red pepper, vitamin C from the jalapeño and red pepper, and fiber from the beans and avocado (not to mention just about every other ingredient). Get ready to add this zestful chili to your recipe rotation!

Serves 4 **Prep time** 15 minutes **Cooking time** 20 minutes

1 yellow onion, chopped

1 medium carrot, chopped

1 red bell pepper, stemmed, seeded, and chopped

3 garlic cloves, minced

2 jalapeños, seeded and minced, optional

2 teaspoons reduced-sodium tamari or coconut aminos

2½ tablespoons chili powder

1 tablespoon ground cumin

2 teaspoons dried oregano

1 14.5-ounce can of diced tomatoes

1½ cups fresh or canned pumpkin puree

2 to 3 cups unsalted or low-sodium vegetable broth

3 cups home-cooked or canned black beans, drained and rinsed

2 to 4 tablespoons freshly squeezed lime juice

Garnish

Sliced green onion, to taste

Avocado cut into ½-inch cubes, to taste

2 to 4 tablespoons pepitas

Freshly chopped cilantro to taste, optional

1. In a large stockpot over medium-high heat, cook the onions, carrots, and red pepper until the onions are translucent, about 3 to 5 minutes. Add 1 to 2 tablespoons of water as needed to deglaze the pan.

2. Mix in the garlic, jalapeños, tamari, chili powder, cumin, and oregano until well combined.

3. Add the tomatoes, pumpkin, 2 cups of broth, and beans. Mix well.

4. Turn down the heat and let simmer for about 15 minutes, stirring occasionally. Add more broth as needed to reach desired consistency.

5. Turn off the heat and add 2 tablespoons of lime juice. Taste for additional lime juice as desired.

6. Spoon into bowls and add green onion, avocado, pepitas, and cilantro.

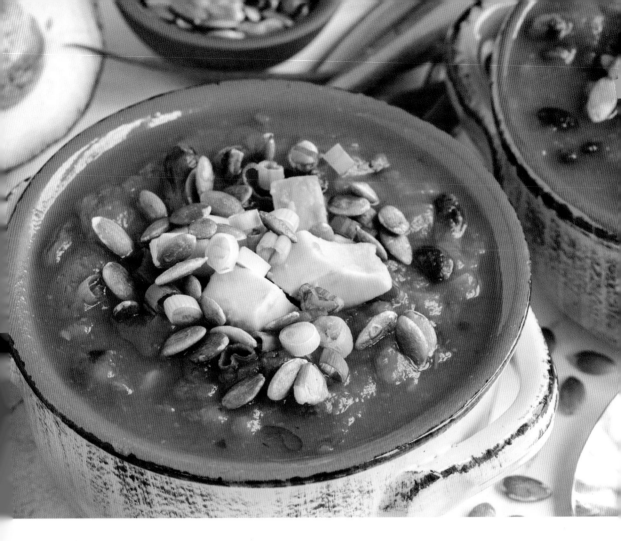

CHEF'S NOTES

Substitutions

Use white or red onion in place of yellow onion.

Use another colorful bell pepper in place of red bell pepper.

Substitute serrano pepper in place of jalapeño pepper.

Instead of pureed pumpkin, use pureed butternut squash.

Substitute kidney beans, pinto beans, or other beans of choice in place of black beans.

Prep Ahead

Cook homemade beans ahead of time and store them in an airtight container in the refrigerator for up to 5 days (or freeze them for up to 1 month).

Storage

Store leftovers in an airtight container in the refrigerator for up to 5 days or freeze them for up to 1 month.

SAVORY VEGAN GUMBO WITH OKRA

Plant-based foods can create similar flavor and texture profiles to just about any traditional meat-based dish. In fact, in our humble opinion, the plant-based versions are even better—especially since they leave you feeling vibrant, energized, and well. This legendary dish has a rich history in New Orleans that includes a mix of cultures in southern Louisiana. Gumbo derives from a West African word for "okra." It can be made with meat, seafood, or simply veggies.

Serves 4 **Prep time** 20 minutes **Cooking time** 6 hours

1 cup yellow or white onion, chopped

5 garlic cloves, minced

2 ribs celery, chopped

1 cup red bell pepper, stemmed, seeded, and chopped

3 cups home-cooked or canned red beans, drained and rinsed

14.5 ounces canned diced tomatoes

2 cups unsalted or low-sodium vegetable broth

2 bay leaves

¼ cup fresh parsley, chopped

2 teaspoons dried oregano

1 teaspoon onion powder

½ teaspoon garlic powder

2 teaspoons ground paprika

1 cup okra, sliced into ½-inch pieces

2 tablespoons arrowroot powder or organic cornstarch

½ teaspoon salt, optional

¼ teaspoon ground black pepper, optional

4 cups cooked brown, black, or red rice

Crushed red pepper flakes, to taste

1. Add all ingredients down to and including the okra to a 4- or 6-quart slow cooker.

2. In a small bowl, add the arrowroot powder and 2 tablespoons of water. Whisk into a slurry and add to the slow cooker.

3. Cook on the low heat setting for 6 hours or the high heat setting for 3 hours.

4. Add salt and pepper, if desired. Taste and boost any flavors you prefer (more salt, garlic powder, paprika, etc.).

5. Spoon onto warm rice and top with red pepper flakes, if desired.

CHEF'S NOTES

Substitutions

Use red onion or shallots in place of white or yellow onion.

Instead of red bell pepper, use yellow or orange.

Instead of canned tomatoes, use about 2 cups of chopped fresh red tomatoes.

Storage

Store leftovers in an airtight container in the refrigerator for up to 5 days or freeze them for up to one month.

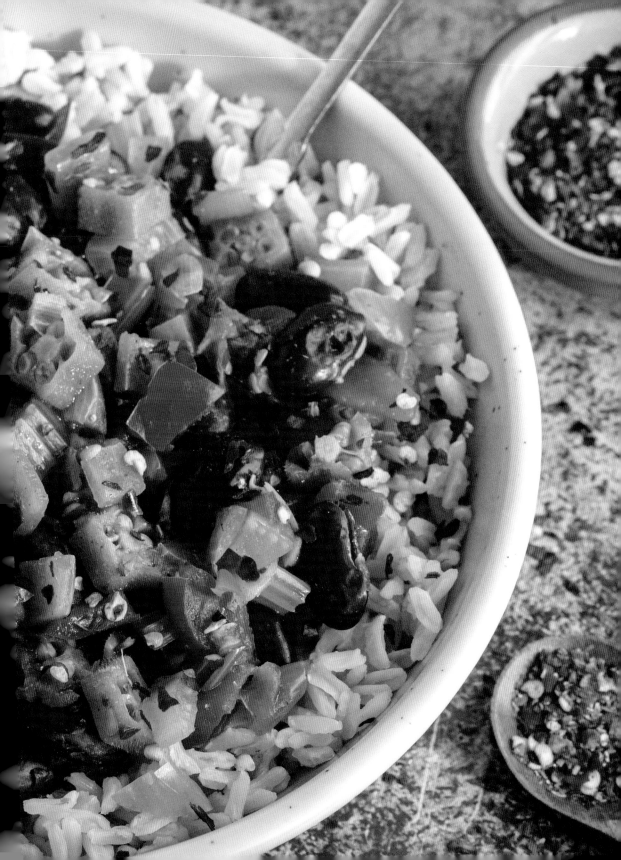

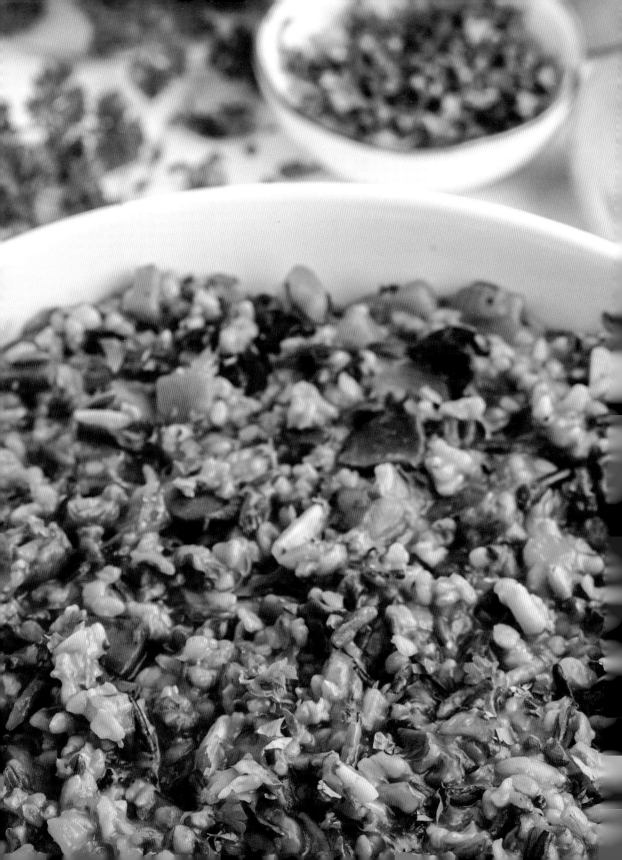

SENSATIONAL SIDES

SLOW-COOKED RAINBOW COLLARDS

Whether you're on the fence about collard greens or have yet to give them a try, this dish may move you into the collard lover camp. A tad bit smoky, with a whole lot of flavor and loads of nutrition, this dish will leave you asking for more and wondering why on earth collards haven't been a staple in your diet (until now).

Serves 4 **Prep time** 15 minutes **Cooking time** 2 hours

1 small red onion, diced

1 cup orange bell pepper, stemmed, seeded, and diced

1 cup yellow bell pepper, stemmed, seeded, and diced

1 cup cherry or grape tomatoes, halved

1½ tablespoons tomato paste

1 tablespoon coconut aminos or reduced-sodium tamari

1 teaspoon smoked paprika

¼ teaspoon salt, optional

1 bunch collard greens, stems removed and thinly sliced

½ cup unsalted or low-sodium vegetable broth

1 tablespoon apple cider vinegar

1. If your slow cooker has a sauté option, set it for 5 minutes, add the onions, orange and yellow peppers, and tomatoes, and sauté them for 5 minutes, stirring occasionally. Add 1 to 2 tablespoons of water as needed to deglaze the pot.

2. Stir in the tomato paste, coconut aminos, smoked paprika, and optional salt.

3. Add the collards and vegetable broth. Stir well, cover, and set to cook on low for 2 hours.

4. If your slow cooker doesn't have the sauté option, simply add all the ingredients except for the apple cider vinegar, and set the slow cooker to cook on low for 2 hours.

5. Once the collards are finished cooking, stir in the apple cider vinegar.

6. Taste and adjust seasoning as desired.

CHEF'S NOTES

Substitutions

Substitute Swiss chard or kale (stems removed) in place of collards.

Instead of red onion, use white or yellow onion.

Use any colorful bell peppers you'd like.

Use white vinegar or sherry vinegar in place of apple cider vinegar.

Storage

Store leftovers in an airtight container in the refrigerator for up to 5 days.

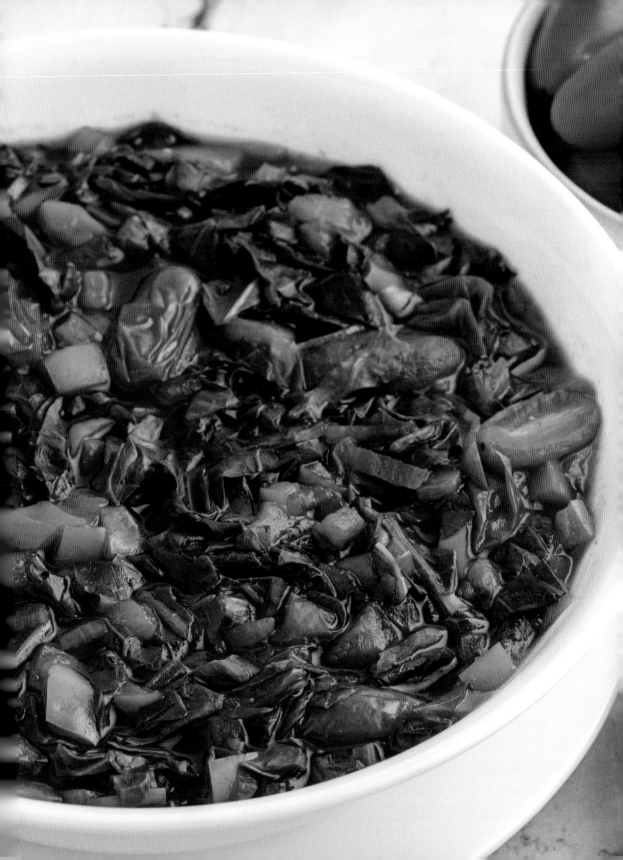

HERBACEOUS WILD RICE AND MUSHROOM STUFFING

Slow cooking wild rice with aromatics, herbs, and mushrooms creates the most exquisite tastes and depths of flavor. Don't own a slow cooker? No problem! Preparing this dish on the stovetop (see Chef's Notes for instructions) still creates the most delectable flavors for your palate and sensational aromas throughout your home while delivering plentiful nutrition to your body.

Serves 4 **Prep time** 15 minutes **Cooking time** 2 hours

1 yellow or white medium onion, chopped

2 medium carrots, chopped

2 ribs celery, chopped

4 garlic cloves, minced

4 cups cremini, button, portobello, or shiitake mushrooms, sliced

1 tablespoon fresh sage, minced

1 tablespoon fresh thyme, minced

¼ teaspoon salt, optional

¼ teaspoon ground black pepper, optional

2 cups dry wild rice

6 cups unsalted or low-sodium vegetable broth

2 cups spinach, chopped

⅓ cup dried unsweetened, unsulfured cranberries, optional

⅓ cup slivered almonds, optional

2 tablespoons fresh parsley, minced

1. For stovetop instructions, see the Chef's Notes.

2. If your slow cooker doesn't have a sauté option, then simply skip that step, add all the ingredients to the pot, and set it to cook per the instructions below.

3. In your slow cooker or Instant Pot, press the sauté button and set the time for 5 minutes. Sauté the onion, carrots, celery, and garlic for 5 minutes, stirring occasionally.

4. Add the mushrooms, sage, thyme, and optional salt and pepper, plus 2 to 3 tablespoons of water to deglaze the pot. Stir and sauté for another 2 minutes. Add the rice and vegetable broth.

5. Set your slow cooker or Instant Pot to high for 2 hours or low for 4 hours.

6. Once the rice is tender, turn off the slow cooker and stir in the spinach until it's wilted.

7. Stir in the cranberries and almonds, if using.

8. Taste and adjust seasoning as desired. Sprinkle parsley on top.

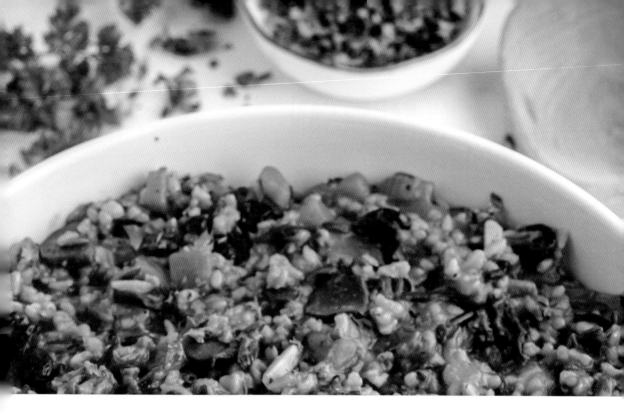

CHEF'S NOTES

Substitutions

Use shallots in place of onion.

Substitute organic black or red rice for wild rice.

Substitute another whole grain of choice in place of rice such as farro or wheat berries. Note the cooking time may be longer with hardier grains.

Substitute another leafy green for spinach, like collards, kale, or Swiss chard.

Instead of cranberries, use raisins.

Substitute sunflower or pumpkin seeds in place of almonds.

Stovetop Instructions

In a large stockpot on medium-high heat, cook the onion, celery, and carrots for 3 to 4 minutes or until the onions are translucent. Stir in the garlic and cook for 1 minute.

Add the mushrooms, sage, thyme, and salt and pepper, plus 1 to 2 tablespoons of water as needed to deglaze the pot. Stir and cook for an additional 2 minutes. Add the rice and broth, bring to a boil, then cover and let them simmer for 40 to 45 minutes or until the rice is tender.

Check the rice halfway and three-quarters of the way through to ensure you don't need more broth or water. Remove from the heat and stir in the spinach. Fold in the cranberries and almonds and sprinkle with parsley.

Storage

Store leftovers in an airtight container in the refrigerator for up to 7 days or freeze them for up to one month.

GARLICKY PARMESAN BROCCOLI

This simple-to-make and flavorsome side includes a true superstar in the plant kingdom: broccoli! The broccoli alone brings lots of nutrients, including sulforaphane, vitamin C, and fiber. Adding a bit of nutty and seedy "parmesan" elevates this side to the next level in both nutrition and flavor. Save the extra parmesan to use on dishes throughout the week!

Serves 2 **Prep time** 10 minutes **Cooking time** 10 minutes

Walnut Parmesan

¾ cup raw, unsalted walnuts, chopped

¼ cup raw, unsalted sunflower seeds

¼ teaspoon garlic powder

¼ teaspoon onion powder

2 tablespoons nutritional yeast

¼ teaspoon salt, optional

Broccoli

6 cups broccoli florets cut into 1- to 2-inch pieces

¼ cup unsalted or low-sodium vegetable broth

5 garlic cloves, minced

1 to 2 squeezes fresh lemon juice

¼ teaspoon salt, optional

Ground black pepper to taste, optional

1. Make the parmesan: Add all the ingredients to a food processor and blend until the walnuts and sunflower seeds are mealy. Important: Don't overblend or you'll end up with parmesan butter!
2. Taste and adjust flavors as desired (more onion, garlic, or nutritional yeast).
3. Steam the broccoli: Bring 24 to 32 ounces of water to a boil.
4. Add the broccoli to a colander (or steam basket) and place it on top of the boiling water. If using a colander, carefully place a lid on top of the colander to keep in the steam.
5. Steam the broccoli for 5 to 6 minutes, depending on your preference for tenderness.
6. In the meantime, heat the vegetable broth in a large stovetop pan on medium-high heat. Add the garlic. Stir and let cook for 1 to 2 minutes.
7. Stir in the broccoli and cook it until the vegetable broth has evaporated, about 1 to 2 minutes.
8. Add a squeeze of lemon juice and optional salt and pepper.
9. Sprinkle 1 to 2 tablespoons of walnut parmesan on top of each serving.

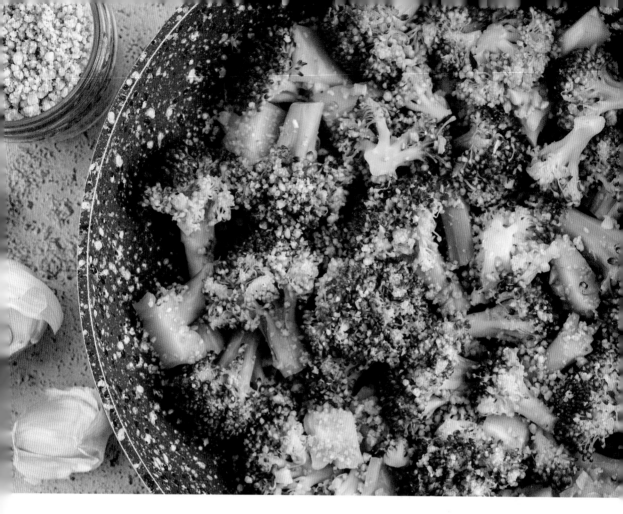

CHEF'S NOTES

Substitutions

Use cauliflower in place of the broccoli.

Instead of walnuts, try almonds or cashews for the parmesan.

Use 1 cup of walnuts total to replace the sunflower seeds in the parmesan.

Use onion granules and/or garlic granules in place of onion and garlic powder (in the parmesan), but know that you might need to use a little more of the granules to reach the same flavor intensity.

Keep It Nut Free

Replace the walnuts with 1 cup total of sunflower seeds.

Prep Ahead

Make the parmesan ahead of time and store it in the refrigerator for up to 2 weeks.

Storage

Store leftovers in an airtight container in the refrigerator for up to 2 weeks or freeze for up to one month.

WARM AND EARTHY HERBED LENTILS

Lentils deliver all the benefits of other legumes, but without the need for soaking first. Warm lentils mixed with fresh rosemary and healing garlic will bring feelings of well-being and comfort when served as a delicious side to a plant-based meal, a tasty addition to green salads, a fun topping on whole grain bread, or a satisfying snack all by themselves.

Serves 4 **Prep time** 10 minutes **Cooking time** 5 minutes

½ cup unsalted or low-sodium vegetable broth

½ cup tomatoes, diced

6 garlic cloves, thinly sliced

2 teaspoons fresh rosemary, minced

2 cups home-cooked or canned brown or green lentils, drained and rinsed

1½ tablespoons freshly squeezed lemon juice

2 tablespoons fresh basil chiffonade

¼ teaspoon salt, optional

¼ teaspoon ground black pepper, optional

Crushed red pepper flakes to taste, optional

1. Heat a large pot on medium-high. Add the vegetable broth, tomatoes, garlic, and rosemary. Turn down the heat to a simmer, stirring often, until the liquid is mostly reduced, about 3 to 5 minutes.
2. Stir in the lentils, then remove from the pot from the heat.
3. Add the lemon juice and fold in the basil until tender.
4. Add salt, black pepper, and crushed red pepper to taste, if desired.
5. Serve as part of a meal, as an appetizer with whole grain bread, or by itself as a snack!

CHEF'S NOTES

Substitutions

For the tomatoes, use any homegrown or organic tomato of choice.

Use fresh thyme or oregano in place of the fresh rosemary.

In place of basil, use parsley or chives.

Prep Ahead

Cook the lentils ahead of time and store them in an airtight container in the refrigerator for up to 5 days (or in the freezer for up to 30 days). Start with approximately 1 cup of dry lentils (plus 3 cups of water) to yield a little over 2 cups when cooked.

Storage

Store leftovers in an airtight container in the refrigerator for up to 5 days or freeze them for up to 30 days.

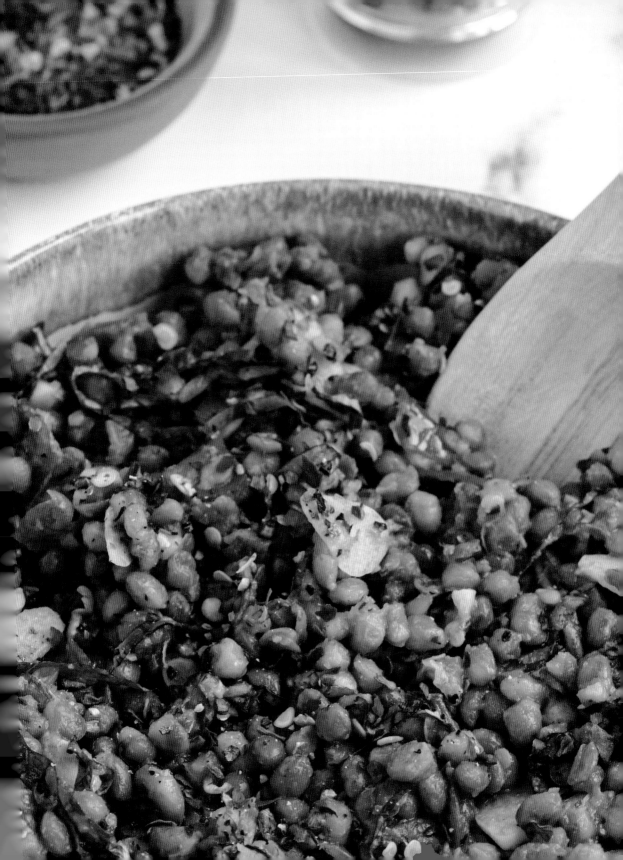

SUBLIME SWEET POTATO MINI DROP BISCUITS

Get ready for these butter- and oil-free biscuits that are perfectly crispy on the outside and moist on the inside. These drop biscuits are made with wholesome plant-based ingredients like sweet potato, plant-based yogurt, and oat flour. Serve them at your next holiday dinner party with a little brushing of maple syrup or date paste and, trust us, your guests will be wowed. Tip: Make extra!

Serves 6 **Prep time** 10 minutes **Cooking time** 18 minutes

Wet Ingredients

⅓ cup plain, unsweetened plant-based milk

1 tablespoon apple cider vinegar

¾ cup cooked and mashed sweet potato, skin removed

¼ cup plain, unsweetened, full-fat almond or cashew yogurt

3 tablespoons pure maple syrup

Dry Ingredients

1 cup oat flour

¼ cup almond flour

2 teaspoons baking powder

½ teaspoon baking soda

½ teaspoon salt

1. Preheat the oven to 450°F and line a baking sheet with parchment paper.

2. In a small bowl, mix the milk and apple cider vinegar and set aside.

3. In a medium bowl, combine the sweet potato, yogurt, and 1 tablespoon of the maple syrup or date paste (reserve the remaining 2 tablespoons for later). Mix well and set aside.

4. In a large mixing bowl, combine all the dry ingredients, then form a well in the center.

5. Slowly add the buttermilk to the center, then mix with the dry ingredients. It should be a bit lumpy.

6. Add the sweet potato mixture and stir to combine. You don't want this batter to be super smooth—a little lumpy is A-OK. It should be a wet mixture but not runny.

7. Drop heaping tablespoons of dough onto the baking sheet. They're going to be rough and coarse around the edges, so don't worry about making them into a ball or flattening them out like a biscuit. They also won't rise much, if at all, so it's okay to space them closely. You should have approximately 18 bite-sized biscuits.

8. Bake for 18 minutes or until the edges are golden brown and crispy. Brush the tops with the remaining maple syrup or date paste.

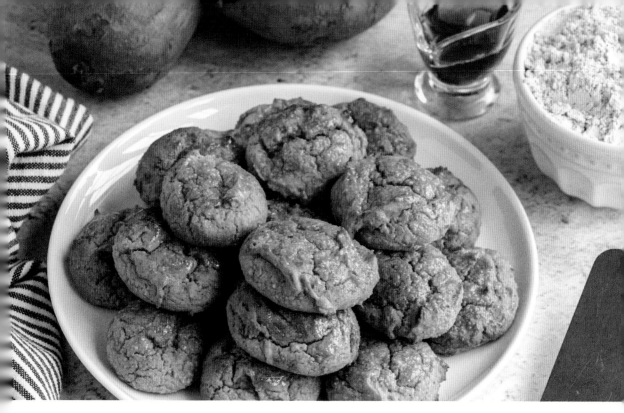

CHEF'S NOTES

Substitutions

Use organic whole wheat flour in place of oat flour.

Whole-Food Sweetener

Use date paste in place of maple syrup.

Prep Ahead

Prepare the sweet potatoes ahead of time by cooking and storing them in an airtight container in the refrigerator for up to 4 days.

Various Ways to Cook Sweet Potatoes

Boil: Peel the sweet potatoes, then cut them into 1-inch cubes. In a pot, completely cover them with water. Heat over medium-high heat until boiling and cook for 10 to 12 minutes or until fork-tender. Drain and allow to cool before mashing with a fork or potato masher.

Roast: Preheat the oven to 425°F and line a baking sheet with parchment paper. Peel the sweet potatoes, then cut into 1-inch cubes. Spread them out evenly on the baking sheet. Bake for 30 minutes or until tender.

Steam: Peel the sweet potatoes, then cut into 1-inch cubes. Place water in a pot to a level just below the steamer basket and bring it to a boil. Add the steamer basket with the sweet potatoes. Maintain a steady boil and steam for approximately 15 minutes or until tender.

Storage

Store leftovers in an airtight container in the refrigerator for up to 7 days. Reheat the biscuits in the oven at 425° to 450°F for 5 to 10 minutes.

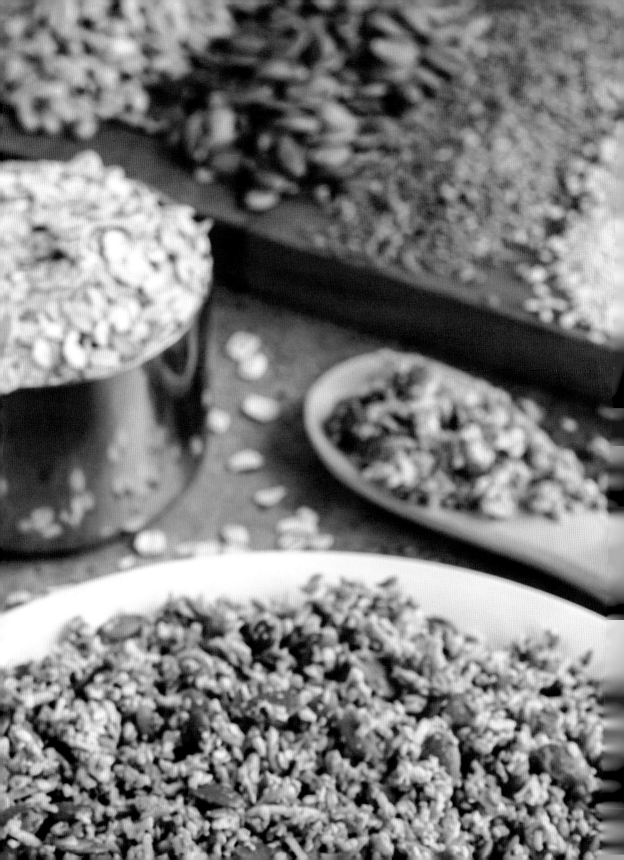

SCRUMPTIOUS SNACKS

ENLIGHTEN ME MATCHA MUFFINS

Experience heightened awareness, better focus, and gentle energy with these satisfying and antioxidant-powered matcha muffins. Make them early in the week and enjoy them all week long as a way to jump-start your mornings or energize your afternoons. Note that if you're caffeine sensitive, these tasty treats do pack a little caffeinated punch. There's about ⅙ teaspoon of matcha per muffin, which is approximately 10 milligrams of caffeine. Not much, but plan accordingly!

Serves 8 **Prep time** 15 minutes **Cooking time** 20 minutes

Chia Egg Substitute

1 tablespoon chia seeds

Dry Ingredients

1 cup oat flour
1 cup rolled oats
2 tablespoons ground flax meal
⅓ cup coconut sugar
2 teaspoons baking powder
¼ teaspoon salt, optional
2 teaspoons unsweetened matcha powder

Wet ingredients

1 cup plain, unsweetened plant-based milk
¼ teaspoon pure vanilla or almond extract
⅓ cup ripe banana, mashed
2 tablespoons tahini

Topping

¼ cup almonds, slivered

1. Preheat the oven to 375°F and line muffin tins with paper cups or use a silicone muffin pan.
2. In a small bowl, whisk together the chia seeds and 3 tablespoons of water. Set aside.
3. In a large bowl, add the dry ingredients and mix until combined.
4. In a medium bowl, add the wet ingredients and stir until combined.
5. Transfer the wet ingredients to the dry and stir well.
6. Fold in the chia egg.
7. Transfer the batter to the muffin cups, filling each about ¾ full. Sprinkle the top of each muffin with slivered almonds, if desired.
8. Bake for 20 minutes or until golden brown.

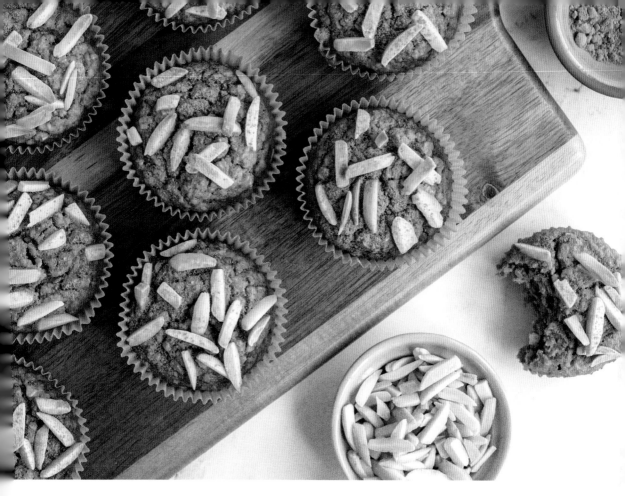

CHEF'S NOTES

Substitutions

Instead of oat flour, use whole wheat flour.

Substitute ¼ of the oat flour with teff flour.

Use ⅓ cup applesauce in place of banana.

Substitute almond butter for tahini.

Whole-Food Sweetener

Substitute date paste for coconut sugar, but add it to the wet ingredients. You will only need ¾ cup plant-based milk instead of 1 cup when you substitute date paste for coconut sugar.

Keep It Nut Free

Omit the almonds and add sunflower seeds, flaxseeds, or another topping of choice.

Storage

Store the muffins in an airtight container in the refrigerator for up to 5 days or freeze them for up to 30 days.

ZESTY CHILI LIME KALE CHIPS

This is a snack that gives back with every bite! Kale chips offer a light crispy crunch, tangy and savory flavor, plenty of fiber, and bountiful phytonutrients. You might be surprised to see the transformation from raw kale leaves that take over the entire baking sheet to what seems like just a handful of crispy kale chips once they're done baking! If you're making these for more than two people or want extra for snacking later, consider doubling the recipe. You'll either need four baking sheets or use the same two baking sheets for two rounds of baking.

Serves 2 **Prep time** 5 minutes **Cooking time** 25 minutes

1 tablespoon tahini

1 tablespoon freshly squeezed lime juice

1 teaspoon chili powder

1 teaspoon garlic powder

4 cups curly or lacinato kale, stemmed with the leaves torn into pieces

1 to 2 pinches of salt, optional

1. Preheat the oven to 250°F and line two baking sheets with parchment paper.
2. In a large bowl, add the tahini, lime juice, chili powder, and garlic powder. Mix well.
3. Add the kale and lightly massage the kale into the lime and spice blend. You'll want the leaves just slightly wilted, so massaging for 15 to 30 seconds will do.
4. Place the kale on the prepared baking sheets in a single layer. Pieces that are overlapping won't dry. Sprinkle 2 pinches of salt onto the kale, if desired.
5. Bake for 20 to 25 minutes or until the kale is dried and crispy. Serve right away or cool completely before storing.

CHEF'S NOTES

Substitutions

In place of kale, use another hardy leafy green such as mustard, collards, or Swiss chard.

Instead of lime juice, use apple cider vinegar or balsamic vinegar.

In place of garlic powder, use onion powder.

Storage

Store the kale chips in a container with the lid slightly open for up to 3 days. Note that leftover kale chips won't be as crispy, so it's best to eat them straight out of the oven!

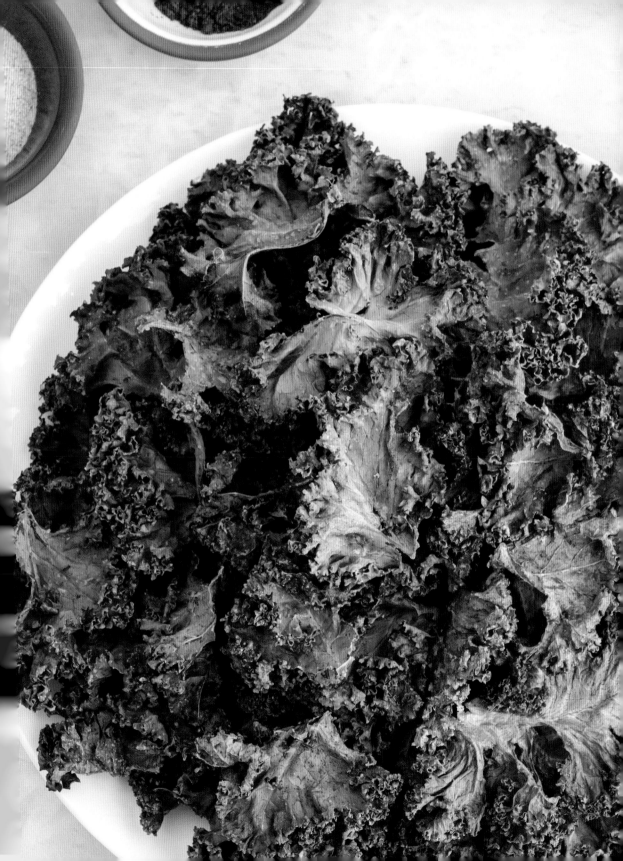

CRISPY MISO ONION CHICKPEAS

A combination of onion granules, organic miso, and reduced-sodium tamari gives these chickpeas plenty of savory flavor, while baking them until crispy gives them that fulfilling crunch for snacking. What's more, fiber and protein-rich chickpeas can help keep you satisfied and energized throughout the day!

Serves 2 **Prep time** 5 minutes **Cooking time** 40 minutes

1 teaspoon mellow white or chickpea miso

1 tablespoon reduced-sodium tamari or coconut aminos

½ teaspoon onion granules or onion powder

2 cups home-cooked or canned chickpeas, drained, rinsed, and dried

1. Preheat the oven to 400°F and line a baking sheet with parchment paper.
2. Whisk the miso, tamari, and onion granules in a medium bowl until the miso is dissolved.
3. Add the chickpeas and stir until they are coated in the miso mixture.
4. Spread the chickpeas evenly on the baking sheet and bake them for 40 minutes, tossing halfway through.
5. Allow them to cool for 5 to 10 minutes (they'll get crispier as they cool!).

CHEF'S NOTES

Substitutions

Instead of chickpeas, use another white bean of choice.

Substitute garlic powder in place of onion powder.

Prep Ahead

Prepare homemade chickpeas ahead of time and store them in an airtight container in the refrigerator for up to 3 days (or freeze them for up to 30 days). Reheat them at 400°F for 10 to 15 minutes before using them.

Storage

Store leftover chickpeas in an airtight container at room temperature for up to 2 days. To make them crispy, reheat them at 375° to 400°F for 5 to 10 minutes.

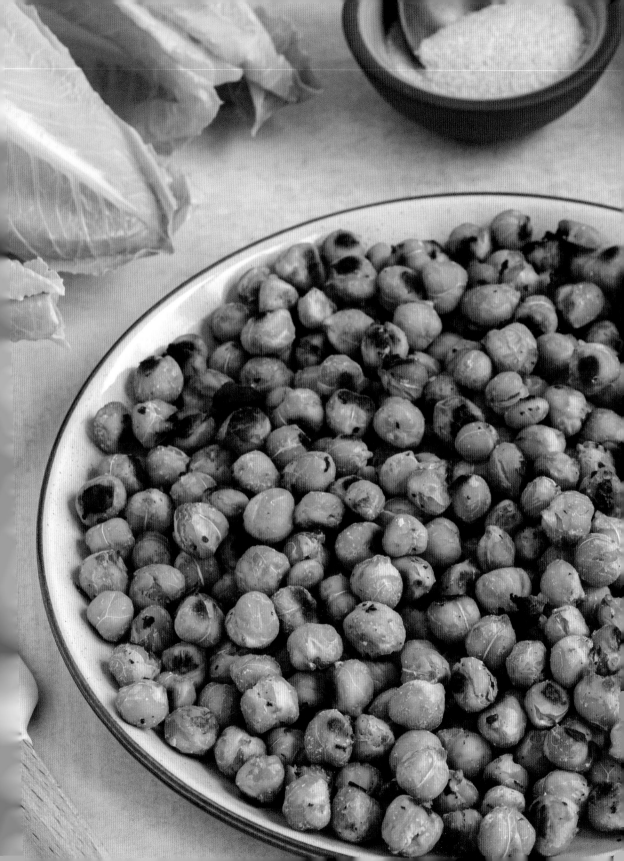

SWEET AND SAVORY SPICED PECANS

These snacking treats come with a warning: their sweet and savory flavor plus perfectly crunchy texture will keep you coming back for more! Pecans fit the superfood category with their plant-based protein, healthy fat, and abundant phytonutrient content, making them an ideal sustainable and nourishing snack. Sweet and Savory Spiced Pecans also add the most incredible flavor and texture to salads and grain bowls. You can also use them as a topping on sweet potatoes and roasted vegetable dishes.

Serves 8 **Prep time** 5 minutes **Cooking time** 15 minutes

2 cups raw and halved pecans
3 tablespoons pure maple syrup
1 teaspoon vanilla extract
1 teaspoon ground cinnamon
1 pinch ground nutmeg
¼ teaspoon salt, optional

1. Preheat the oven to 350°F.
2. Add all the ingredients except for the pecans to a medium bowl. Mix well.
3. Add the pecans to the bowl and mix well.
4. On a parchment-lined baking sheet, spread out the pecans evenly.
5. If desired, sprinkle just a touch of salt over the pecans. You could also add a little more maple syrup, cinnamon, or spice at this point, if you especially love particular flavors.
6. Bake for 15 minutes, tossing/turning the pecans halfway through to ensure even baking.
7. Remove the sheet from the oven and let the pecans cool. They'll get crispy as they cool.

CHEF'S NOTES

Substitutions

Walnuts, pistachios, or some combination of the three nuts would be delicious!

Whole-Food Sweetener

Use orange juice in place of the maple syrup, and note that the final result might be less crispy.

Make It Spicy

Before baking, sprinkle a dash of cayenne pepper on top of the pecans.

Storage

Store the pecans in an airtight container at room temperature for up to 2 weeks, in the refrigerator for up to 1 month, or in the freezer for up to 3 months.

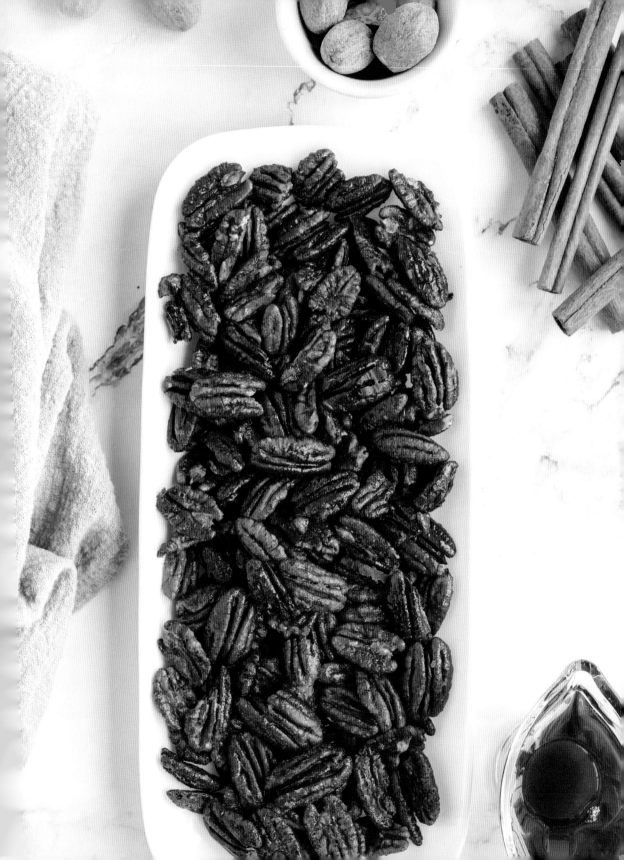

SUPER SEEDY GRANOLA

A nut-free take on traditional granola that is just as tasty, crunchy, and nutritious! This granola is yummy by itself as a snack, or you can enjoy it as a cereal with plant-based milk or on top of plant-based yogurt for some crunch. The superfood seeds are packed with zinc, magnesium, and iron.

Serves 4 **Prep time** 5 minutes **Cooking time** 20 minutes

½ cup raw, unsalted pumpkin seeds
½ cup raw, unsalted sunflower seeds
½ cup brown or golden flaxseeds
¼ cup hulled sesame seeds
1 cup unsweetened shredded coconut
1 cup uncooked rolled oats
¼ cup pure maple syrup
1½ teaspoons pure vanilla extract
1 teaspoon ground cinnamon
2 pinches of salt, optional

1. Preheat the oven to 325°F.
2. Add all the seeds and shredded coconut to a large bowl. Mix well.
3. Add the oats to a food processor and pulse until they have a meal-like consistency. Stir the oats into the large bowl with the seed mixture.
4. Add the maple syrup, vanilla extract, ground cinnamon, and optional salt. Mix well until the dry ingredients are moistened.
5. Spread the mixture out evenly on a parchment-lined baking sheet.
6. Bake for 20 minutes or until golden brown, tossing halfway through. Let cool for 10 minutes before enjoying. It will get crispier upon cooling.

CHEF'S NOTES

Substitutions

Use any seeds you like for this! If there is a particular seed you don't like or cannot find, then skip it and add more of your favorite.

Whole-Food Sweetener

You can use date paste in place of the maple syrup. However, the final result may not be as crispy, and you may need to thin the date paste with water to a syrup
consistency in order for it to stick to the entire seed mixture.

Baking Tips

Oven temperatures can differ. Check the granola halfway through as you're tossing to determine how quickly it's cooking. It can burn, so keep an eye on it!

Storage

Once the granola is fully cool, store it in an airtight container at room temperature for up to 10 days or refrigerate it for up to 1 month. Note, if you use date paste as the sweetener, it'll only keep in the refrigerator for up to 1 week.

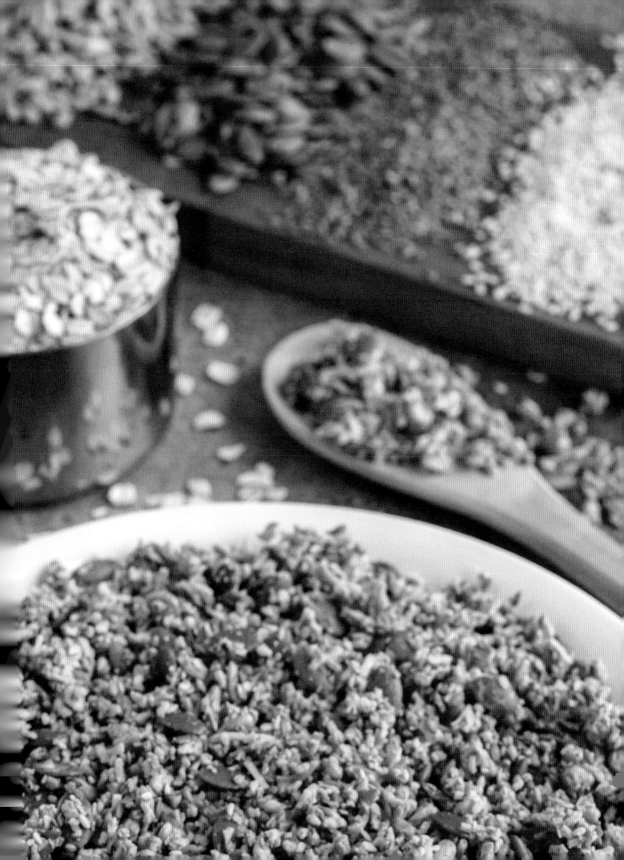

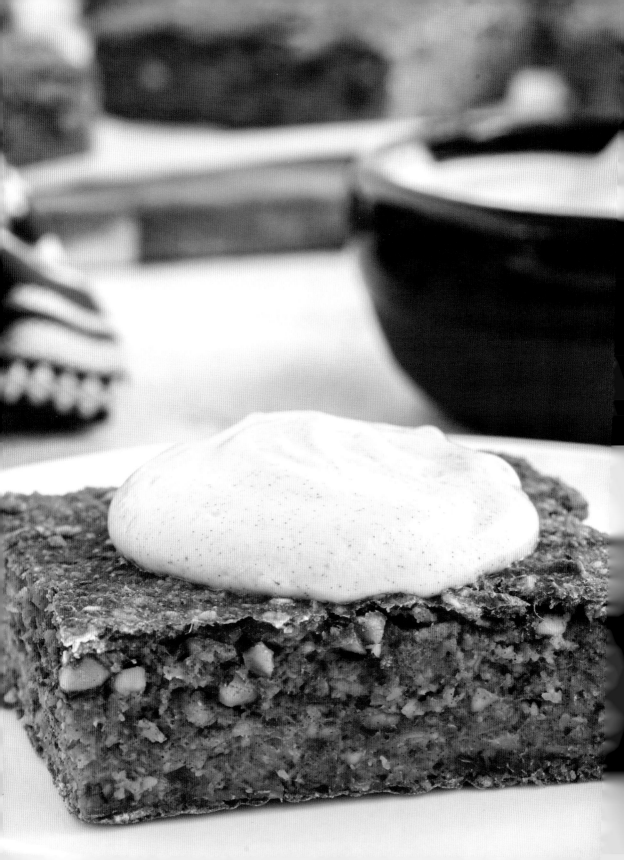

DIVINE DESSERTS

OH-SO-SWEET GREEN TEA PISTACHIO NICE CREAM

With lots of antioxidants in the green tea, prebiotic fiber in the banana, and plant-based protein in the pistachios, this is an ice cream that you can feel good about as you savor each refreshing taste. Coconut cream adds extra creaminess, but rest assured that it'll still be super creamy (thanks to the banana) if you choose to omit it. Add some fresh berries on top for even more superfood goodness!

Serves 2 **Prep time** 5 minutes **Cooking time** none

2 small ripe bananas

½ cup coconut cream, optional

2 teaspoons unsweetened matcha powder

¼ cup pistachios, shelled and chopped

1. Add the bananas, coconut cream (if using, see Chef's Notes), and matcha powder to a blender or food processor. Blend until smooth and creamy.
2. Transfer to a freezer-safe container. Stir in the pistachios.
3. Freeze for 1 to 2 hours, stirring every 20 minutes for the first hour.
4. To serve, let the ice cream sit at room temperature until it's soft enough to divide into bowls. Top with more pistachios, if desired.

CHEF'S NOTES

Substitutions

If you're sensitive to caffeine, substitute moringa powder or acai powder for the matcha powder.

Saturated-Fat-Free Version

If you're watching your cholesterol levels, omit the coconut cream.

Storage

Store in an airtight container in the freezer for up to 2 weeks.

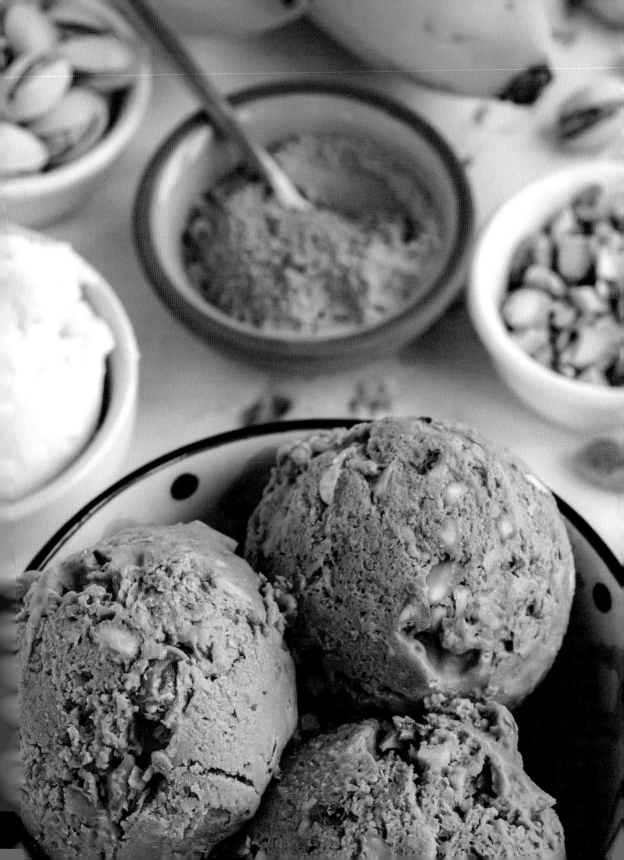

BRIGHT AND FRUITY BLUEBERRY LEMON BARS

These bars might seem indulgent at first bite, but what you're experiencing is the power of plant-based foods and their healthy decadence! These treats are slightly sweet with a bit of tartness and include all the elements to make your kitchen smell incredible and your body feel fabulous. And they're not just for dessert—enjoy them for breakfast or as a midafternoon snack.

Serves 6 **Prep time** 15 minutes **Cooking time** 40 minutes

Filling

3 cups fresh or frozen blueberries
¼ cup pure maple syrup
2 tablespoons chia seeds
½ cup freshly squeezed lemon juice
2 tablespoons lemon zest
2 tablespoons arrowroot powder or corn starch

Dough

1 cup rolled oats
2 tablespoons hulled hemp seeds
1 cup almond meal
1 cup oat flour
1 teaspoon baking powder
2 pinches of salt, optional
⅓ packed cup mashed ripe banana
¼ cup pure maple syrup
¼ cup unsweetened plant-based milk
1 teaspoon pure vanilla extract

1. Preheat the oven to 375°F. Line a loaf pan or 8-inch square baking dish with parchment paper.
2. Make the filling: Add the blueberries, maple syrup, chia seeds, lemon juice, and lemon zest to a small saucepan. Cook over medium heat, stirring occasionally, for 6 to 8 minutes or until the filling is bubbly and resembles pourable blueberry jam. (Optional: mash half the blueberries with a spatula or leave them all whole if you like more texture.)
3. Make the arrowroot slurry by combining the arrowroot powder with 2 tablespoons of water in a small bowl. Mix until the arrowroot is dissolved.
4. Stir the arrowroot slurry into the blueberries until the mixture thickens (about a minute). Remove from the heat and set aside.
5. In a large mixing bowl, add the oats, hemp seeds, almond meal, oat flour, baking powder, and salt. Stir well to combine.
6. In a small bowl, add the mashed banana, maple syrup, milk, and vanilla. Mix well.
7. Add the wet banana mixture to the dry ingredients. Mix well to form a dough.
8. Spread ⅔ of the dough in the parchment-lined baking dish.

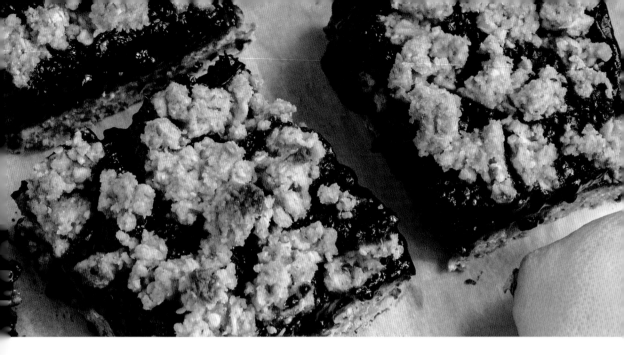

9. With a spatula, spread the filling evenly on top of the dough.

10. Crumble the remaining ⅓ of the dough on top of the filling. (The crumble will be moist, so it may not exactly "crumble" on top. Basically, you're placing pieces of the crumble along the top, and it may not cover the entire dish. That's okay!)

11. Bake for 30 minutes or until the crumble top is golden brown. Let the bars sit for 10 minutes.

12. Once cool, remove the berry bake by pulling the parchment paper out from the baking dish and transferring it to a cutting board. Cut into 2 x 2-inch bars.

CHEF'S NOTES

Substitutions

Use another berry of choice in place of blueberries.

Use another fruit of choice like cubed apples or pears in place of blueberries.

Whole-Food Sweetener

Use date paste in place of maple syrup.

Berries

Frozen organic wild blueberries are small and have a higher water content than fresh berries, making the bars extra gooey. Your final filling consistency may depend on the type of berries you use.

Prep Ahead

Make the filling ahead of time and store it in an airtight container in the refrigerator for up to 2 days.

Storage

Store leftovers in an airtight container in the refrigerator for up to 5 days or freeze them for up to 30 days.

SUMMERTIME STRAWBERRY RHUBARB CRISP

If you're a fan of strawberry rhubarb pie, then you're going to love this simple-to-prepare crisp. Strawberries and rhubarb get their pretty red color from compounds called anthocyanins, which have been shown to cultivate a healthy gut, lower blood pressure, decrease cholesterol, and reduce the risk of certain types of cancer. The crispy topping is packed with fiber and plant-based protein from the oats and the almonds. Can we get a cheer for plant-based foods that offer loads of nutrition in one scrumptious dessert?

Serves 6 **Prep time** 15 minutes **Cooking time** 30 minutes

Fruit

4 cups strawberries, stemmed and cut into quarters

4 cups rhubarb, cut into ½-inch pieces

⅓ cup pure maple syrup

½ cup arrowroot powder or corn starch

2 tablespoons freshly squeezed lemon juice

⅛ teaspoon salt, optional

Topping

1 cup rolled oats

1 cup almond meal

1 cup oat flour

1 teaspoon baking powder

2 pinches of salt, optional

⅓ packed cup mashed banana

¼ cup pure maple syrup

¼ cup unsweetened plant-based milk

1 teaspoon pure vanilla extract

1. Preheat the oven to 350°F and line a baking sheet with parchment paper.
2. In a large bowl, toss together the strawberries, rhubarb, maple syrup, arrowroot powder, lemon juice, and optional salt. Spread out the fruit evenly on the parchment-lined baking sheet. Set aside.
3. Make the topping: In the same large mixing bowl that you used for the fruit, add the oats, almond meal, oat flour, baking powder, and optional salt. Stir well to combine.
4. In a small bowl, add the mashed banana, maple syrup, plant-based milk, and vanilla. Mix well.
5. Add the wet banana mixture to the dry ingredients. Mix well to form a dough.
6. Crumble the dough on top of the strawberry mixture. (The crumble will be moist, so it may not exactly "crumble" on top. Basically, you're placing pieces of the crumble along the top, and it may not cover the entire sheet. That's okay!)
7. Bake for 30 minutes or until the top is golden brown.

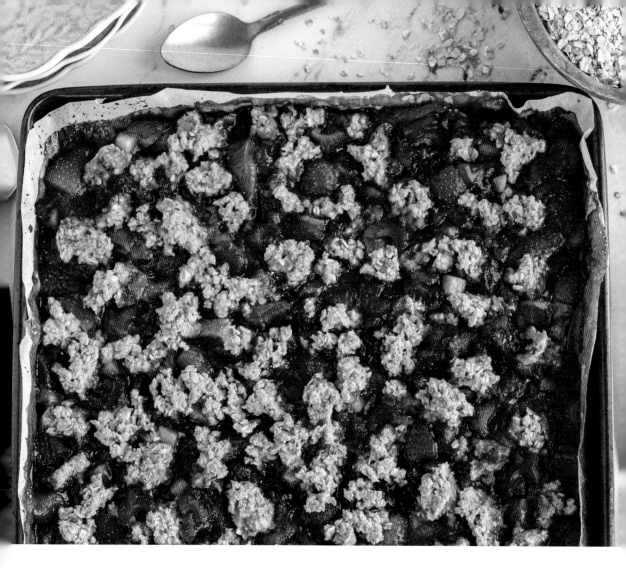

CHEF'S NOTES

Substitutions

Substitute any two fruits (or one single) fruit that is in season or that you have on hand for the strawberries and rhubarb.

Substitute ⅓ cup unsweetened applesauce for banana.

Whole-Food Sweetener

Use date paste in place of maple syrup.

Prep Ahead

Prepare the topping ahead of time and store in an airtight container in the refrigerator for up to 2 days.

Storage

Store leftovers in an airtight container in the refrigerator for up to 5 days. Reheat the crisp in the oven at 350°F for 10 to 15 minutes.

VELVETY CHOCOLATE BERRY DESSERT CUPS

The combination of rich dark chocolate with tart, fruity raspberries is simply divine—these two superstar plant-based foods really were made for each other! Plus, they combine their individual nutrient profiles to create a treat that is packed with the antioxidants that make them good for your health. If getting creative in the kitchen is your idea of fun, then this recipe is for you!

Serves 5 (makes 20 cups) **Prep time** 25 minutes **Cooking time** 10 minutes

Raspberry Puree

2 cups fresh or frozen raspberries

2 tablespoons pure maple syrup

1 tablespoon freshly squeezed lemon juice

½ teaspoon vanilla extract

1 pinch salt, optional

1 tablespoon arrowroot powder or organic cornstarch

Chocolate Cups

9 ounces fair-trade or direct trade 85% dark chocolate

1. Line a mini muffin tin with 20 small paper liners (we used 1.37-inch mini paper baking cups).

2. Make the raspberry puree: Heat a small pan on medium-high heat. Add 1 cup of raspberries (reserve the other cup for later), maple syrup, lemon juice, ¼ cup of water, vanilla, and optional salt. Bring to a boil, then simmer, stirring occasionally, until the puree thickens and reduces by about 30 percent (about 5 to 7 minutes).

3. Meanwhile, mix the arrowroot powder and 1 tablespoon of water in a small bowl to make a slurry.

4. Once the raspberry puree has reduced, stir in the arrowroot slurry until the puree thickens to a jam-like consistency, about 30 seconds. Turn off the heat and set the pan aside to cool.

5. Meanwhile, melt the chocolate in a double boiler. (Alternatively, you could melt the chocolate in the microwave using a microwave-safe bowl in 30-second increments, stirring in between, until the chocolate has completely melted.)

6. Using a teaspoon, add the melted chocolate to each of the liners to line the bottom. Gently tap the muffin pan on the countertop to even out the chocolate and remove any air bubbles. Place the pan in the freezer for 5 minutes to allow the chocolate to harden.

7. Once the chocolate has hardened, place ½ to ¾ teaspoon of the raspberry puree (make sure it's cool) into the center of each chocolate cup. Spoon more melted chocolate over the filling (about 1½ teaspoons of chocolate) to fully cover the top and the sides. Add 1 whole raspberry to the center of each cup. Refrigerate until the chocolate hardens, about 30 minutes, or freeze the cups for 15 minutes. Store them in the refrigerator until you are ready to eat.

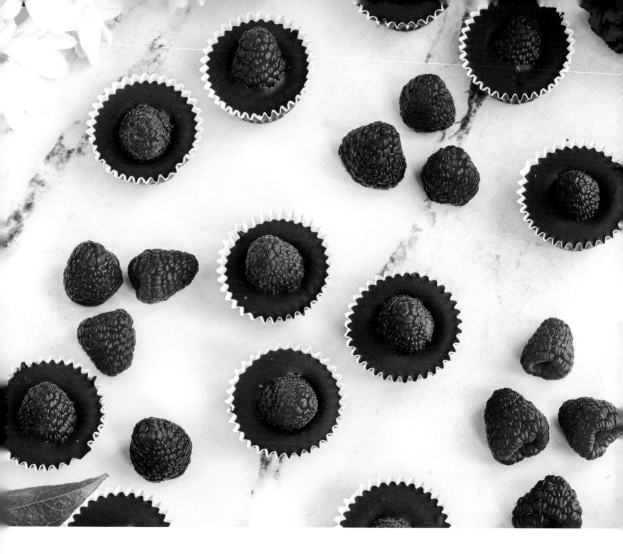

CHEF'S NOTES

Substitutions

Use another berry in place of raspberries, like organic strawberries or blueberries.

Substitute a different percentage of dark chocolate. We recommend greater than 70%, and always make sure it's fair-trade or direct-trade.

Substitute 3 tablespoons date paste in place of maple syrup.

Prep Ahead

Make the raspberry puree ahead of time and keep it in an airtight container in the refrigerator for up to 5 days.

Storage

Store the chocolates in an airtight container in the refrigerator for 5 to 7 days.

SWEET VITALITY CARROT CAKE

Did someone say cake can create health and vitality? Fresh turmeric and ginger have been shown to decrease inflammation through their phytonutrients, curcumin, and gingerol, respectively. Prebiotic fiber in the oats feeds healthy bacteria in the gut. And the carotenoids in carrots are free radical scavengers. This zesty and luscious cake is perfect on its own, but if you've always loved the cream cheese frosting on traditional carrot cake, we've included a creamy, plant-based alternative!

Serves 8 **Prep time** 15 minutes **Cooking time** 45 minutes

Vanilla Cashew Cream

1 cup raw, soaked cashews (see Chef's Notes)
½ cup unsweetened plant-based milk
¼ cup date paste
1½ teaspoons vanilla extract
1 pinch salt, optional

Chia Egg

1 tablespoon chia seeds
3 tablespoons water

Cake Batter

1½ cups unsweetened plant-based milk
½ cup pitted and soaked Medjool dates, see Chef's Notes

½ cup mashed ripe banana
2 teaspoons vanilla extract
1 tablespoon apple cider vinegar
1¾ cups oat flour
1 cup rolled oats
2 teaspoons baking powder
1 teaspoon baking soda
2 teaspoons ground cinnamon
2 tablespoons fresh ginger, grated
1 tablespoon fresh turmeric, grated
1 teaspoon ground nutmeg
2 pinches of ground cloves
¼ teaspoon salt, optional
⅛ teaspoon ground black pepper, optional
1½ cups carrots, shredded
¾ cup walnuts, chopped

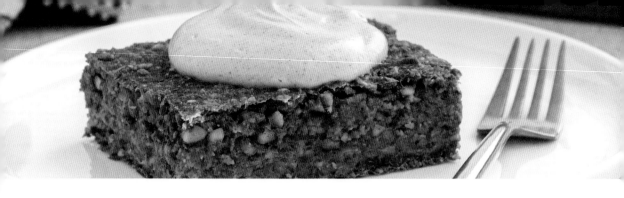

1. Preheat the oven to 350°F.
2. Drain the soaked cashews (see Chef's Notes). Blend the cashews, milk, date paste, vanilla, and salt in a blender or food processor until smooth.
3. Taste and boost any additional flavor of your choice (more dates for sweetness, more vanilla, etc.) or add additional milk if you'd like a thinner consistency. Set aside.
4. In a small bowl, make the chia egg substitute by mixing the chia seeds and 3 tablespoons of water. Set aside.
5. Once the dates have been soaked, drain them. In a blender, blend the dates, milk, vanilla, banana, and apple cider vinegar until smooth. Set aside.
6. In a large mixing bowl, combine the oat flour, rolled oats, baking powder, baking soda, cinnamon, ginger, turmeric, nutmeg, cloves, salt and pepper, and shredded carrots.
7. Transfer the wet ingredients to the dry ingredients. Mix well.
8. Fold in the chia egg. Stir in the walnuts.
9. Transfer the mixture to a parchment-lined 8- or 9-inch square baking dish or into individual ramekins (sprayed lightly with cooking spray). Bake for 40 to 45 minutes or until crispy and golden on top.
10. Once cool, spread the Vanilla Cashew Cream on top, if desired.

CHEF'S NOTES

Substitutions

In place of date paste in the Vanilla Cashew Cream, use maple syrup. Note that maple syrup will give the cream a slightly thinner consistency.

In place of oat flour, use almond flour, but note that you may need to reduce the amount of plant-based milk by approximately 25 percent.

Instead of walnuts add pecans.

Use ½ teaspoon of ground ginger and ½ teaspoon of ground turmeric in place of fresh ginger and fresh turmeric.

Make Carrot Muffins

Line muffin tins with paper liners and fill to the top. Bake at 350°F for 20 to 25 minutes or until golden brown on top. Makes approximately 18 muffins.

Prep Ahead

Soak the dates and keep in an airtight container in the refrigerator for up to 48 hours. Alternatively, soak the dates in warm water for 10 minutes before using.

Make the Vanilla Cashew Cream ahead of time. Soak the cashews for 4 to 6 hours before preparing the cream. Store the cashews in an airtight container in the refrigerator for up to 4 days.

Storage

Store leftover carrot cake in an airtight container in the refrigerator for up to 5 days or in the freezer for up to 30 days.

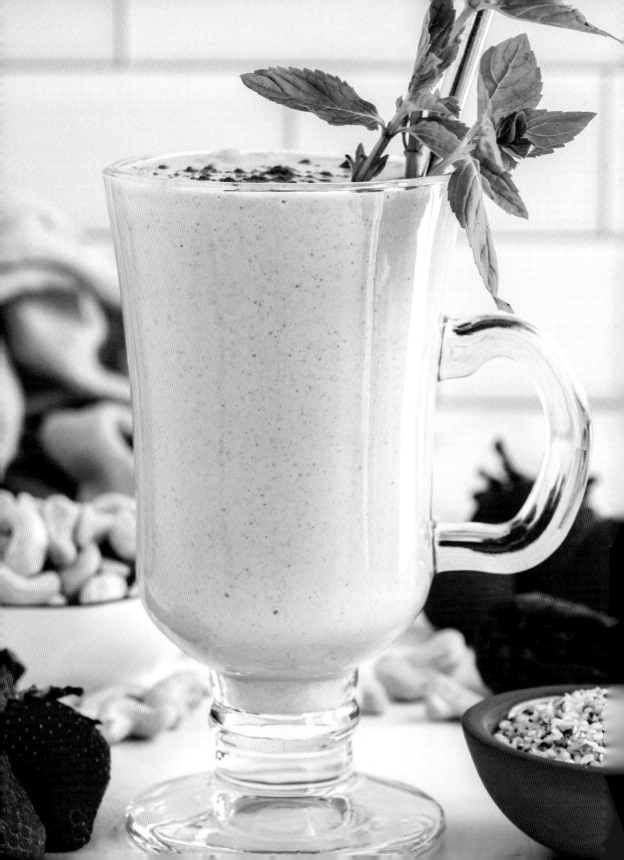

DYNAMIC DRINKS

GOLDEN GLOW LEMONADE

Refreshing yet invigorating and rejuvenating—that's how this healing beverage feels as you're sipping and savoring it. Ginger and turmeric have anti-inflammatory compounds that heal at the cellular level. Use fresh ginger and turmeric if you're able to find them, as they really do have more zing. Ground turmeric and ginger are lovely options as well!

Serves 2 **Prep time** 10 minutes **Cooking time** 20 minutes

¼ cup ginger, peeled and roughly chopped

¼ cup turmeric, peeled and roughly chopped

1 tablespoon whole black peppercorns

¼ cup freshly squeezed lemon juice

½ cup unsweetened 100% pineapple juice

2 tablespoons fresh mint leaves, optional

1. Steep the tea: Add 3 cups of water along with the ginger, turmeric, and peppercorns to a medium pot. Heat on medium-high until boiling, then lower the heat to simmer for 20 minutes.
2. Allow the tea to cool before straining the tea into a pitcher or 32-ounce mason jar.
3. Add the lemon and pineapple juices and stir. If you're using a jar with a lid, tighten the lid and shake well.
4. Taste and boost the sweetness (pineapple juice) or tartness (lemon juice), depending on your preference.
5. Enjoy your lemonade at room temperature or pour it over ice. Garnish with fresh mint leaves and pineapple chunks (on skewers if you'd like to get fancy!).

CHEF'S NOTES

Substitutions

Use organic apple juice, mango juice, or orange juice in place of pineapple juice.

Instead of fresh turmeric, mix 1 teaspoon of ground turmeric into the lemonade-pineapple mixture.

Instead of fresh ginger, mix 1 teaspoon of ground ginger into the lemonade-pineapple mixture.

Add Other Flavors

Steep hibiscus along with the ginger, turmeric, and peppercorns for deep color, more nutrition, and a tart berry flavor.

Muddle berries into the juice.

Make it a green tea by steeping green tea with the ginger and turmeric.

Make it spicy by adding a dash of cayenne pepper.

Rather than using as a garnish, steep the mint with the ginger and turmeric.

Make a Spritzer

Add 8 ounces of carbonated water to 8 ounces of the lemonade.

Storage

Store leftovers in a pitcher, covered, or mason jar in the refrigerator for up to 7 days.

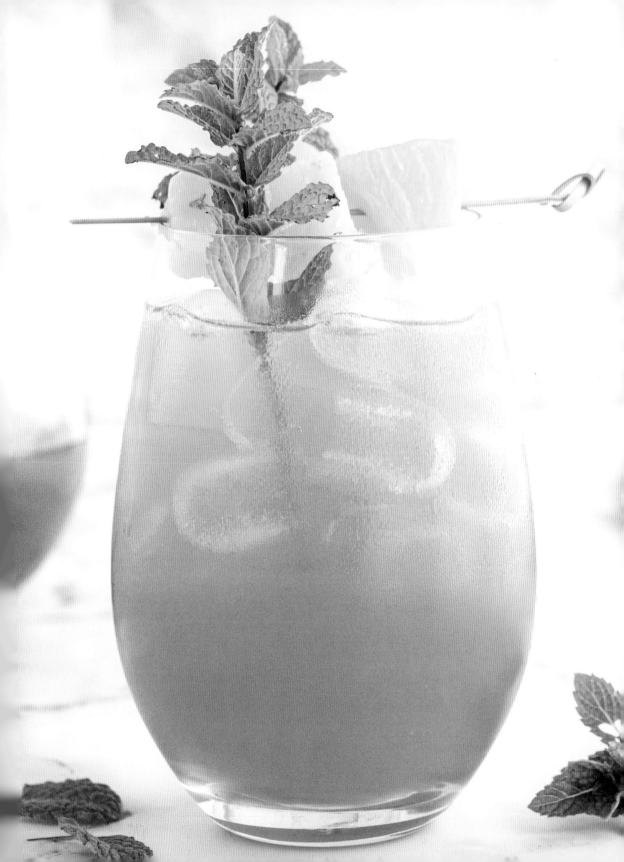

COOL AS A CUCUMBER MATCHA REFRESHER

Cool As a Cucumber Matcha Refresher is for those times when you need something hydrating, stimulating, and energizing. Matcha offers an antioxidant punch, while cucumbers provide lots of hydrating water, and mint helps to open the senses. This recipe calls for pineapple juice, but if you prefer whole foods, whole fresh pineapple would work as well!

Serves 2 **Prep time** 5 minutes **Cooking time** none

2 cups unwaxed, skin on cucumber, chopped (or peeled cucumber if waxed)

¼ cup mint leaves, chopped

¼ cup freshly squeezed lemon juice

¼ cup unsweetened 100% pineapple juice

2 teaspoons unsweetened matcha powder

2 sprigs mint

1. Add the cucumber, mint leaves, lemon juice, pineapple juice, matcha, and 1 cup of water to a blender. Blend until smooth, about 2 to 3 minutes.
2. Pour into two 12-ounce glasses filled with ice (if desired).
3. Garnish with a mint sprig and enjoy!

CHEF'S NOTES

Substitutions

For the cucumber, you can use Persian or English.

Use lime juice in place of lemon juice, if desired.

Use orange juice, mango juice, or other juice of your choice in place of pineapple juice.

Whole-Food Sweetener

Use whole fresh or frozen pineapple in place of pineapple juice. Note that you may need to add a bit more water to reach the desired consistency.

No-Pulp Variation

If you blend this juice until smooth, you should have very little pulp. However, if you want it even smoother, strain the juice before pouring over ice.

Storage

Store leftover juice in the refrigerator in a mason jar or pitcher for up to 5 days.

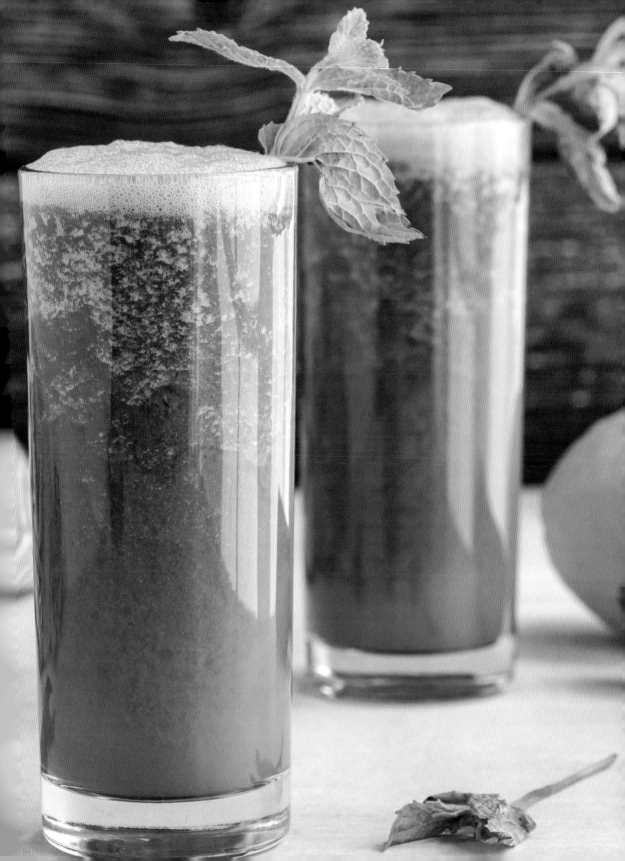

SOUL-SOOTHING GOLDEN MILK

Soothe your soul while supporting optimal health as you sip and savor this creamy and earthy golden milk. Relish it in the morning as a replacement for coffee or enjoy it as a calming beverage before bedtime, preparing your body for deep sleep.

Serves 1 **Prep time** 2 minutes **Cooking time** 5 minutes

8 ounces unsweetened plant-based milk of choice
1 teaspoon tahini
1 teaspoon vanilla extract
½ teaspoon ground turmeric
½ teaspoon ground cinnamon
¼ teaspoon ground ginger
1 dash ground black pepper
1 dash ground cloves
1 dash ground nutmeg

1. Add the plant-based milk, tahini, and vanilla to a small saucepan. Heat on medium-high until hot and steaming (don't let it scorch or boil, though), stirring until the tahini completely dissolves (this shouldn't take more than 1 minute).
2. While the milk is heating, combine the spices in a small bowl and mix them until well blended.
3. Once the milk and tahini mixture is hot, turn off the burner and add the spice mixture to the saucepan with the milk. Whisk until all the spices have dissolved.
4. Pour into your favorite mug and enjoy!

CHEF'S NOTES

Substitutions

Instead of ground spices, use whole cinnamon, cloves, ginger, and turmeric by simmering them in the plant-based milk for about 10 minutes and straining them out when ready to serve.

Make It Creamier

Unsweetened, organic soy milk will result in the creamiest consistency among the most common kinds of plant milk.

Consider adding another teaspoon of tahini to make it creamier, but know that it will impart a slight tahini flavor to the milk—which is great if you love tahini!

Use almond butter or another nut or seed butter in place of the tahini. They'll make the drink a little creamier and add a bit of natural sweetness without sugar.

Consider using 8 ounces of canned light coconut milk in place of 8 ounces of the other plant-based milk.

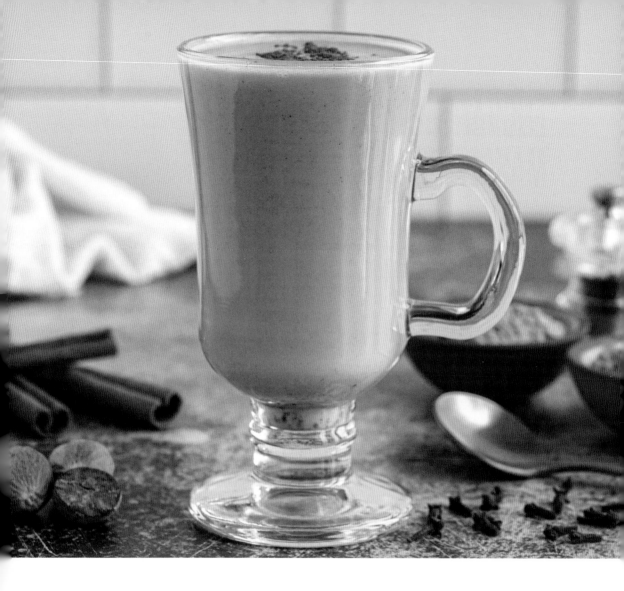

Add Some Sweetness

The tahini gives this drink a little natural sweetness. If you'd like a bit more, add a teaspoon of pure maple syrup.

If you have a blender handy, you could allow the finished milk to cool slightly before transferring it to a blender, adding 1 or 2 dates, and blending well for some natural sweetness. This will also ensure that the spices are well blended with the milk. Transfer the blended mixture back to the stovetop pot to warm through before pouring it into your mug.

Storage

Store leftovers in an airtight container or mason jar in the refrigerator for up to 3 days.

ENCHANTING MASALA CHAI

Warm and nourishing chai may be the perfect antidote to cold temperatures, internal stress, or the winter blues. The first step to fostering comfort and calm is simply the process of making chai. This beverage uses whole healing spices—if you're able, take time to notice their beautiful shapes, aromas, and textures as you add them to the water. Slowly infusing the spices into the water will create the spicy, invigorating masala flavors. Plant-based milk is added for a little creaminess, and the amount of sweetness is up to you!

Serves 2 **Prep time** 5 minutes **Cooking time** 15 minutes

2 cinnamon sticks

2 star anise

12 whole cloves

3 cardamom pods, cracked open

8 peppercorns, optional

1 tablespoon fresh ginger, sliced

3 to 4 tablespoons loose leaf rooibos tea (see Chef's Notes)

2 cups unsweetened, plant-based milk

Coconut sugar to taste, optional

1. Add 4 cups of water and the spices, from the cinnamon sticks to the ginger, to a medium pot. Bring to a boil, then simmer for 10 minutes to concentrate the spices (the liquid will reduce by half).
2. Turn the heat down to low, add the rooibos tea, and let it steep for 4 to 5 minutes.
3. Strain the tea and spices through a fine-mesh strainer into a large pitcher or jar.
4. Heat the milk in the same pot until it just starts to boil.
5. Combine the milk with the tea.
6. Divide the chai between two mugs. Add coconut sugar or another sweetener of choice as desired.

CHEF'S NOTES

Substitutions

If you can't find whole spices, use the following ground ratios to make your masala spice blend:
1 teaspoon ground cinnamon
1¼ teaspoons ground ginger
¼ teaspoon ground cloves
½ teaspoon ground nutmeg
¼ teaspoon ground cardamom
¼ teaspoon ground allspice
⅛ teaspoon ground black pepper

If you can tolerate (and want) caffeine, use black tea in place of rooibos tea.

Sugar-Free Version

Chai is typically sweetened, but it's not necessary to do so if you prefer a sugar-free beverage.

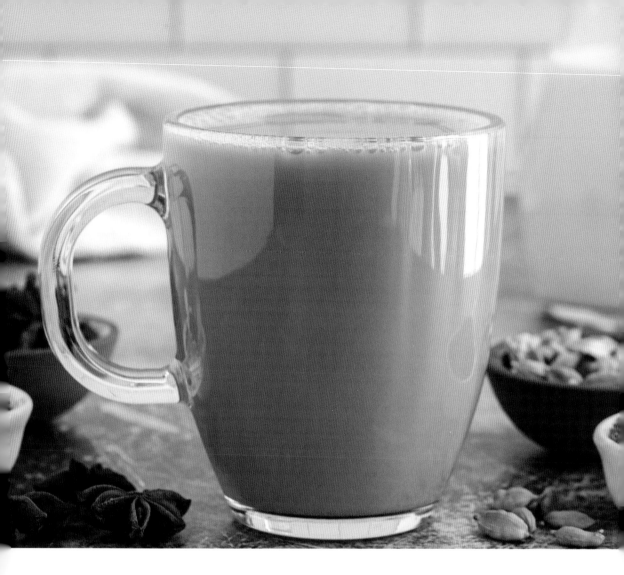

Spice Options

Masala spice is really a personal preference. If you prefer less spice, then use less ginger. If you don't like licorice flavor, then omit the star anise. The flavor blend can easily be modified to your taste.

Add Adaptogens

Add ½ to 1 teaspoon of maca, ashwagandha, or cordyceps to each cup for additional hormone balancing.

Storage

Store leftover chai in an airtight container or mason jar in the refrigerator for up to 3 days.

MINDFULNESS MOMENT MATCHA TEA

Start your day energized or give your afternoon slump a boost with this calming yet invigorating tea. Matcha can support steady energy, a gentle sense of awareness, and improved focus while turmeric supports immune health and fights inflammation. Matcha and turmeric are true superstars when it comes to plants that nourish!

Serves 2 **Prep time** 5 minutes **Cooking time** 5 minutes

12 ounces unsweetened plant-based milk

2 teaspoons unsweetened matcha powder

½ teaspoon ground turmeric

¼ teaspoon ground cinnamon

2 dashes nutmeg

2 dashes ground black pepper

1. Heat 12 ounces water and the milk in a small saucepan until you see steam, but don't let it boil (this curdles the milk and is not good for matcha's nutrients).
2. Meanwhile, combine the turmeric, cinnamon, nutmeg, and pepper in a small bowl.
3. Once the water and milk mixture is hot, turn off the heat and add the matcha and the spice mixture.
4. Whisk until all the powder is dissolved. It may take a vigorous whisking for 1 to 2 minutes. Alternatively, you could use an immersion blender.
5. Divide the tea between two mugs.

CHEF'S NOTES

Substitutions

Don't have matcha? Steep a green tea bag in 6 ounces of hot (not boiling) water for 2 to 3 minutes while warming 6 ounces of unsweetened, plant-based milk on the stovetop. Once the milk is hot, add the spice blend to it. Pour in the green tea.

Substitute fairly traded cocoa powder for matcha tea to get a similar boost in energy and antioxidants!

Make It Sweeter

If this is your first matcha experience, it might taste a little bitter, but the more you drink it, the less bitter it will taste. Your tastebuds will adjust! You can add 1 teaspoon of maple syrup or coconut nectar to temper the bitterness.

Add one teaspoon of vanilla extract.

If you're using a blender instead of a whisk, add 1 to 2 dates.

Make It Creamier

Omit the water and use 12 ounces of plant-based milk.

Add 4 ounces light coconut cream.

Storage

Store leftovers in an airtight container or mason jar in the refrigerator for up to 3 days.

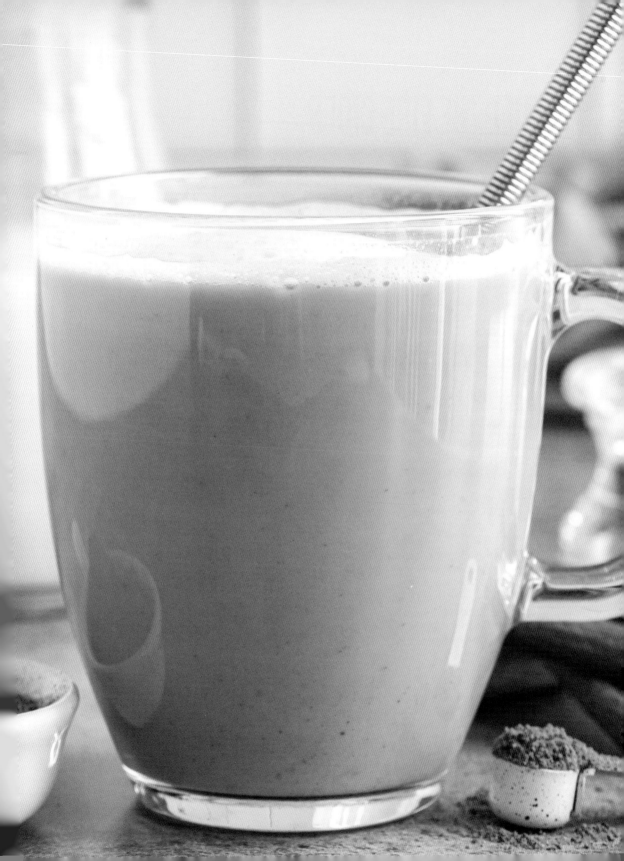

FUEL THE FIRE CIDER

Patience is the name of the game when making Fuel the Fire Cider, and it's very much worth the wait! The ingredients in this beverage all have their own unique phytonutrients that make it an invigorating and healthful tonic. Plus, it's magnificently tasty. Enjoy an ounce a day for immune system support.

Serves 2 **Prep time** 10 minutes (+ 4 weeks) **Cooking time** none

2 tablespoons fresh ginger, minced

2 tablespoons garlic, minced

¼ cup red onion, chopped

2 tablespoons habanero pepper, chopped

1 tablespoon fresh turmeric, minced

1 teaspoon jarred horseradish, with vinegar and salt only

¼ cup lemon zest

1 teaspoon mustard seed

1 teaspoon fennel seed

1 tablespoon fresh rosemary

1 tablespoon whole peppercorns

2 cups apple cider vinegar

1. Add all the ingredients except the apple cider vinegar to a 16-ounce mason jar.

2. Pour the apple cider vinegar over the ingredients until they are completely submerged.

3. Lay a piece of parchment paper over the rim of the jar. Screw the lid tightly in place. Shake well.

4. Let the mixture sit in a dark, cool place for four weeks, shaking once daily.

5. After four weeks, pour the contents into a muslin or cheesecloth-lined colander positioned over a stable pot. Let the cider drain for 30 minutes, then gather the corners of the cloth, twisting and squeezing until all of the liquid is released. When the cider is fully strained, add a touch of pure maple syrup or date nectar if desired and pour the mixture into a sterilized canning jar.

6. Enjoy an ounce of this beverage daily as an invigorating tonic.

CHEF'S NOTES

Substitutions

Use one teaspoon of turmeric powder or ginger powder in place of fresh spices.

Use one teaspoon of dried rosemary in place of fresh rosemary.

If you don't have habanero pepper, you can use jalapeño or a teaspoon of red pepper flakes. If you don't want the spice, simply omit the pepper.

Use white or yellow onion in place of red.

Use ½ teaspoon of freshly grated horseradish root in place of a bottled horseradish.

Storage

Store in a cool, dark place for up to a year, shaking well before using.

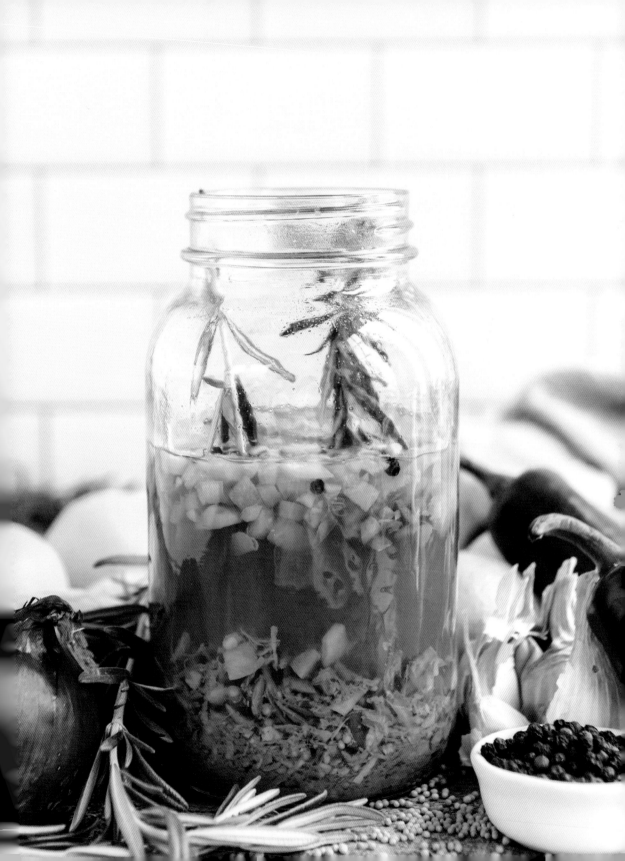

INVIGORATING TROPICAL GREEN SMOOTHIE

Smoothies are definitely a Food Revolution Network team favorite because of their ability to squeeze many superfoods into one fabulous and refreshing drink. This delicious smoothie includes prebiotic fiber (banana), probiotic bacteria (yogurt), colorful phytonutrients (pineapple and kale), and even more fiber from the chia seeds. Kick-start your day or recharge your afternoon with a restorative lift as you savor this power-charged smoothie.

Serves 2 **Prep time** 5 minutes **Cooking time** none

1 cup unsweetened, plant-based yogurt
2 handfuls kale, leaves only
2 cups fresh or unsweetened canned pineapple
1 ripe banana
2 tablespoons chia seeds

1. Add all the ingredients to a blender with 1 cup of water and blend until smooth.
2. Taste and boost with additional ingredients of choice.
3. Add more water as needed to reach desired consistency.

CHEF'S NOTES

Substitutions

Instead of kale, try watercress, mustard greens, or broccoli sprouts.

In place of pineapple, use mango or a combination of the two.

Instead of yogurt, use plant-based kefir.

Storage

Store leftovers in an airtight container in the refrigerator for up to 3 days. Add more water as needed for consistency.

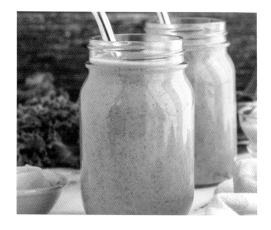

PURPLE PARADISE SMOOTHIE

Naturally sweet blueberries, zesty ginger, and earthy greens make a refreshing and energizing smoothie to revitalize your senses and ignite your soul. Use any greens you have on hand, and if strong-flavored greens are growing in your garden (such as dandelion or kale), balance their bitterness by adding more blueberries for sweetness or ginger for added zing!

Serves 2 **Prep time** 10 minutes **Cooking time** none

1½ cups fresh or frozen blueberries
1 cup romaine lettuce, chopped
1 cup unsweetened, plant-based milk
4 tablespoons rolled oats
1 teaspoon fresh ginger, minced
⅓ teaspoon ground cinnamon

1. Add all ingredients and ice, if desired, to a blender and blend until smooth.
2. Taste and boost with additional ingredients of choice (more greens, berries, ginger, or cinnamon).
3. Divide the smoothie between two serving glasses and top with an additional sprinkle of cinnamon, if desired.

CHEF'S NOTES

Substitutions

Substitute another berry of choice for blueberries, such as strawberries, raspberries, or blackberries.

Substitute hemp seeds in place of oats.

Make It Sweet

Add 1 to 2 pitted dates or 1 to 2 tablespoons of date paste before blending.

Storage

Store leftovers in an airtight container or mason jar for up to 3 days.

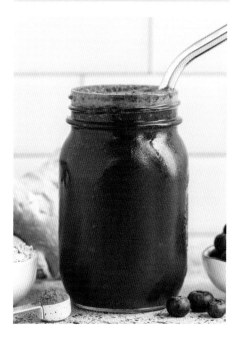

HEMP-TASTIC STRAWBERRY SHORTCAKE SMOOTHIE

Berries are nutritious whether they're fresh or frozen, which means they're available year-round, making them ideal for smoothies. This smoothie is certainly refreshing in the summertime but is also ideal during the winter since strawberries are powered with vitamin C, cashews have lots of zinc, and hemp seeds are a great source of plant-based protein and healthy fats—all nutrients that support year-round healthy living!

Serves 1 **Prep time** 10 minutes **Cooking time** none

1 cup strawberries, sliced, green tops removed
½ cup raw cashews
½ cup rolled oats
2 medium pitted dates
2 tablespoons hulled hemp seeds
1 teaspoon vanilla extract
1 sprig mint, optional
1 dash ground cinnamon, optional

1. Add 1 cup of water and all the ingredients except the mint and cinnamon to a blender and blend on high until the strawberries, cashews, and hemp seeds are completely blended. An immersion blender will also work but might take a little longer.
2. Garnish with a sprinkle of cinnamon, more hemp seeds, and a sprig of mint if desired.

CHEF'S NOTES

Substitutions

Blueberries, blackberries, and/or raspberries could be delicious substitutes for strawberries.

Pecans or walnuts can be used in place of cashews but tend to result in a grittier texture.

Whichever rolled oats you have on hand, quick or old-fashioned, work just fine.

Layer It Up

Add a teaspoon of your favorite superfood powder like spirulina, maca, or moringa to the smoothie.

Add a teaspoon of cinnamon to really ramp up the spice quotient.

Add 1 to 2 tablespoons of chia seeds for crunch and texture (you might need to add a little extra water as well until you get the desired consistency).

Add a tablespoon of cacao powder for a chocolaty berry drink.

Add ½ a banana for a banana-strawberry treat.

Storage

Store leftovers in an airtight container or mason jar in the refrigerator for up to 3 days.

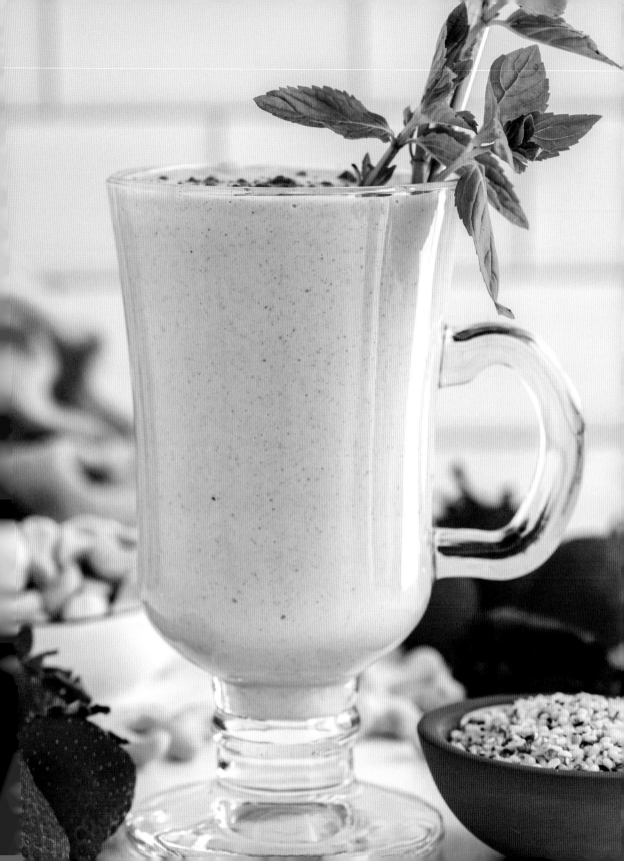

ESPRESSO MY LOVE OF MOCHA SMOOTHIE

Frosty, cool, and sweet, featuring the iconic pairing of espresso and chocolate, this recipe will surely make it into your smoothie rotation. Banana, dates, cacao powder, walnuts, and hemp seeds all provide important trace minerals, such as magnesium, iron, potassium, and copper. Oats, dates, and cacao are also excellent sources of B vitamins, which help to support cellular energy production, making this an ideal smoothie for when you need some pep in your step.

Serves 2 **Prep time** 10 minutes **Cooking time** none

1½ cups unsweetened, plant-based milk

1½ fresh or frozen bananas

½ cup rolled oats

2 tablespoons hulled hemp seeds

¼ cup raw walnuts

1 tablespoon fair-trade or direct-trade cacao or cocoa powder

2 pitted dates

2 to 4 tablespoons brewed espresso

1 to 2 handfuls ice, optional

1. Add all the ingredients, except the ice, to a blender and blend until smooth.
2. Taste and boost flavors with additional ingredients of your choice.
3. Add 1 to 2 handfuls of ice and blend again.
4. Divide between two glasses and sprinkle with cacao or cocoa powder, if desired.

CHEF'S NOTES

Substitutions

Use pecans or cashews in place of walnuts.

For the espresso, use caffeinated or decaffeinated, whichever you prefer.

For a less strong mocha smoothie, or if you don't have an espresso option, add 1 to 2 ounces of coffee in place of espresso.

Espresso-Making Options

Some coffee makers have an espresso option, which is helpful!

To make espresso in a French press, use medium-fine grind. Heat ¾ cup of water until it is hot but not boiling. Add the espresso to the French press, followed by the water. Stir and let stand for 4 minutes before using the espresso in your smoothie.

Keep It Nut Free

Instead of walnuts, use raw sunflower seeds.

Storage

Store leftovers in an airtight container or mason jar in the refrigerator for up to 3 days.

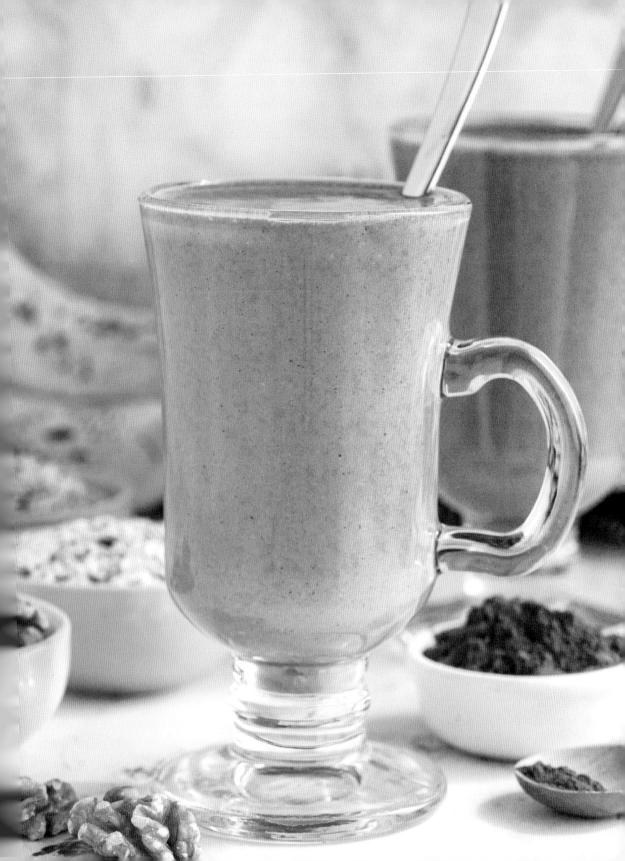

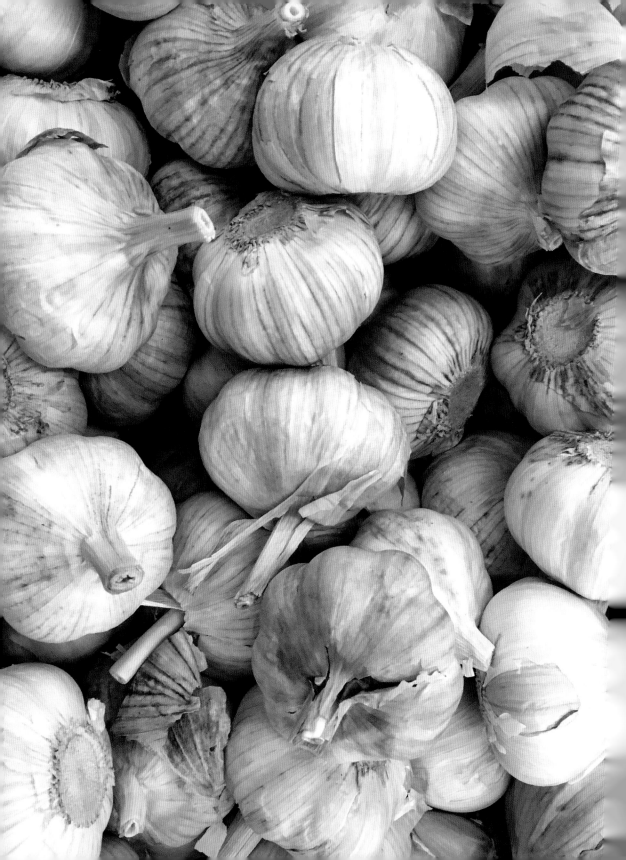

ENDNOTES

Introduction

1. "Adult Obesity Facts," Centers for Disease Control and Prevention, last modified May 17, 2022, https://www.cdc.gov/obesity/data/adult.html.

2. "Leading Causes of Death," Centers for Disease Control and Prevention, last modified September 6, 2022, https://www.cdc.gov/nchs/fastats/leading-causes-of-death.htm.

3. Kate Eller, "These 27 Medical Problems Are Caused by a Poor Diet," health enews, last modified October 24, 2017, https://www.ahchealthenews.com/2017/10/24/27-medical-problems-caused-poor-diet.

4. "Stop Using Antibiotics in Healthy Animals to Prevent the Spread of Antibiotic Resistance," World Health Organization, last modified November 7, 2017, https://www.who.int/news/item/07-11-2017-stop-using-antibiotics-in-healthy-animals-to-prevent-the-spread-of-antibiotic-resistance.

5. Winston Wong, "Economic Burden of Alzheimer Disease and Managed Care Considerations," *American Journal of Managed Care* 26, no. 8 (August 2020): S177–S182, https://www.ajmc.com/view/economic-burden-of-alzheimer-disease-and-managed-care-considerations.

6. Steve Finlay, "GM Is Getting Sick of High Health Care Costs," WardsAuto, last modified March 1, 2004, https://www.wardsauto.com/news-analysis/gm-getting-sick-high-health-care-costs.

7. "US Health Expenditure as Percent of GDP from 1960 to 2021," Statista, last modified January 9, 2023, https://www.statista.com/statistics/184968/us-health-expenditure-as-percent-of-gdp-since-1960.

8. "US Defense Outlays and Forecast as a Percentage of GDP 2000–2032," Statista, last modified September 30, 2022, https://www.statista.com/statistics/217581/outlays-for-defense-and-forecast-in-the-us-as-a-percentage-of-the-gdp.

9. J. Poore and T. Nemecek, "Reducing Food's Environmental Impacts Through Producers and Consumers," *Science* 630, no. 6392 (June 2018): 987–992, https://www.science.org/doi/10.1126/science.aaq0216.

10. "Disrupting Meat," Yale Center for Business and the Environment, last modified October 12, 2016, https://cbey.yale.edu/our-stories/disrupting-meat.

11. "World Hunger Facts," Action Against Hunger, last accessed January 24, 2023, https://www.actionagainsthunger.org/world-hunger-facts-statistics.

Chapter 1

1. Frugé et al., "A Dietary Intervention High in Green Leafy Vegetables Reduces Oxidative DNA Damage in Adults at Increased Risk of Colorectal Cancer: Biological Outcomes of the Randomized Controlled Meat and Three Greens (M3G) Feasibility Trial," *Nutrients* 13, no. 4 (April 2021), doi:10.3390/nu1304122.

2. Ocean Robbins, "What Is Sulforaphane?" Food Revolution Network, last modified December 16, 2020, https://foodrevolution.org/blog/what-is-sulforaphane/.

3. Morris et al., "Nutrients and Bioactives in Green Leafy Vegetables and Cognitive Decline: Prospective Study" *Neurology* 90, no. 3 (2018): e214–e222, doi:10.1212/WNL.0000000000004815.

4. Michael Greger, "Brain-Healthy Food to Fight Aging," *Nutrition Facts*, last modified December 26, 2018, https://nutritionfacts.org/video/brain-healthy-foods-to-fight-aging.

5. "Nutrition Facts: Kale," University of Rochester Medical Center, last accessed January 24, 2023, https://www.urmc.rochester.edu/encyclopedia/content.aspx?contenttypeid=76&contentid=11236-1.

6. "Nutrition Facts: Spinach," University of Rochester Medical Center, last accessed January 24, 2023, https://www.urmc.rochester.edu/encyclopedia/content.aspx?contenttypeid=76&contentid=11463-2.

7. Cooper et al., "Fruit and Vegetable Intake and Type 2 Diabetes," *European Journal of Clinical Nutrition* 66 (2012): 1082–1092, https://doi.org/10.1038/ejcn.2012.85.

8. Blekkenhorst et al., "Cardiovascular Health Benefits of Specific Vegetable Types: A Narrative Review." *Nutrients* 10, no. 5 (May 2018), doi:10.3390/nu10050595.

Chapter 2

1. "White button mushroom phytochemicals inhibit aromatase activity and breast cancer cell proliferation" in J. Nutrition, 2001 Dec;131(12):3288-93 https://pubmed.ncbi.nlm.nih.gov/11739882/

2. Hannah Sentenac, "Why Healing Your Gut (and Keeping Your Gut Happy) Is Essential for Good Health," Food Revolution Network, last modified February 27, 2018, https://foodrevolution.org/blog/best-foods-for-gut-health.

3. Sentenac, "Why You Need Both Probiotics and Prebiotics for Good Gut Health and Overall Wellness (Plus the Best Food Sources)," Food Revolution Network, last modified September 14, 2018, https://foodrevolution.org/blog/probiotics-and-prebiotics.

4. Paul Stamets, "Mushrooms and Mycelium Help the Microbiome," GreenMedinfo, last modified July 27, 2016, https://greenmedinfo.com/blog/mushrooms-and-mycelium-help-microbiome.

5. Ergothioneine is associated with reduced mortality and decreased risk of cardiovascular disease, BMJ Heart, https://heart.bmj.com/content/106/9/691

6. Mushroom Consumption and Incident Dementia in Elderly Japanese: The Ohsaki Cohort 2006 Study; J Am Geriatr Soc. 2017 Jul;65(7):1462-1469, https://pubmed.ncbi.nlm.nih.gov/28295137/

7. The Association between Mushroom Consumption and Mild Cognitive Impairment: A Community-Based Cross-Sectional Study in Singapore, J Alzheimers Dis. 2019;68(1):197-203 https://pubmed.ncbi.nlm.nih.gov/30775990/

8. Ocean Robbins, "Amazing Study: Mushrooms Reduce Breast Cancer by 64%," Food Revolution Network, March 1, 2016, https://foodrevolution.org/blog/how-to-fight-prevent-cancer-with-mushrooms.

9. Twardowski et al., "A Phase I Trial of Mushroom Powder in Patients with Biochemically Recurrent Prostate Cancer: Roles of Cytokines and Myeloid-derived Suppressor Cells for *Agaricus bisporus*–induced Prostate-specific Antigen Responses," *Cancer* 121, no. 17 (September 2015): 2942–2950, https://doi.org/10.1002/cncr.29421.

10.   Ocean Robbins, "The Power of Mushrooms: Nutrition, Benefits, and Risks of Edible Mushrooms," Food Revolution Network, last modified December 11, 2020, https://foodrevolution.org/blog/mushrooms-nutrition-benefits-risks.

11.   Reynolds et al., "Carbohydrate Quality and Human Health: A Series of Systematic Reviews and Meta-analyses," *The Lancet* 393, no. 10170 (February 2019): P434–445, https://www.thelancet.com/article/S0140-6736(18)31809-9/fulltext.

12.   Lindsay Oberst, "Mushrooms Have Stunning Powers to Heal People and the Planet," Food Revolution Network, last modified July 30, 2021, https://foodrevolution.org/blog/health-benefits-of-mushrooms.

Chapter 3

1.   Poulain et al., "Identification of a Geographic Area Characterized by Extreme Longevity in the Sardinia Island: the AKEA study," *Experimental Gerontology* 39, no. 9, (2004): 1423–1429, https://halshs.archives-ouvertes.fr/halshs-00175541/file/2004%20POULAIN%20BZ%20EXP%20GERONT.pdf.

2.   "The World's #1 Longevity Food," Blue Zones, last accessed January 24, 2023, https://www.bluezones.com/2016/06/10-things-about-beans/.

3.   Lanza et al., "High Dry Bean Intake and Reduced Risk of Advanced Colorectal Adenoma Recurrence Among Participants in the Polyp Prevention Trial," *The Journal of Nutrition* 136, no. 7 (2006): 1896–1903, doi:10.1093/jn/136.7.1896.

4.   P. N. Singh and G. E. Fraser, "Dietary Risk Factors for Colon Cancer in a Low-risk Population," *American Journal of Epidemiology* 148, no. 8 (1998): 761–774, doi:10.1093/oxfordjournals.aje.a009697.

5.   Jukanti et al., "Nutritional Quality and Health Benefits of Chickpea (Cicer arietinum L.): A Review," *British Journal of Nutrition* 108, no. S1 (2012): S11–S26, doi:10.1017/S0007114512000797.

6.   Marc P. McRae, "The Benefits of Dietary Fiber Intake on Reducing the Risk of Cancer: An Umbrella Review of Meta-analyses," *Journal of Chiropractic Medicine* 17, no. 2 (2018): 90–96, doi:10.1016/j.jcm.2017.12.001.

7.   Mazza et al., "Impact of Legumes and Plant Proteins Consumption on Cognitive Performances in the Elderly," *Journal of Translational Medicine* 15, no. 1 (May 2017): 109, doi:10.1186/s12967-017-1209-5.

8.   Paula Cohen, "The MIND Diet: 10 Foods that Fight Alzheimer's (and 5 to Avoid)," CBS News, March 30, 2015, https://www.cbsnews.com/media/mind-diet-foods-avoid-alzheimers-boost-brain-health.

9.   Yanni Papanikolaou and Viktor L. Fulgoni, "Bean Consumption is Associated with Greater Nutrient Intake, Reduced Systolic Blood Pressure, Lower Body Weight, and a Smaller Waist Circumference in Adults: Results from the National Health and Nutrition Examination Survey 1999-2002," *Journal of the American College of Nutrition* 27, no. 5 (October 2008): 569-76, doi: 10.1080/07315724.2008.10719740.

10.   Winham, Donna, Andrea M. Hutchins, and Carol S. Johnson, "Pinto Bean Consumption Reduces Biomarkers for Heart Disease Risk," *Journal of the American College of Nutrition* 26, no. 3 (2007): 243–249, doi:10.1080/07315724.2007.10719607.

11.   Polak, Rani, Edward M. Phillips, and Amy Campbell, "Legumes: Health Benefits and Culinary Approaches to Increase Intake," *Clinical Diabetes* 33, no. 4 (October 2015): 198–205, https://doi.org/10.2337/diaclin.33.4.198.

Chapter 4

1.   Michael Greger, "Best Berries," *Nutrition Facts*, last modified January 9, 2012, https://nutritionfacts.org/video/best-berries/.

2.   Khalid et al., "Effects of Acute Blueberry Flavonoids on Mood in Children and Young Adults" *Nutrients* 9, no. 2 (2017): 158, https://doi.org/10.3390/nu9020158.

3. Jessica Maki, "Berries Keep Your Brain Sharp," *The Harvard Gazette*, last modified April 26, 2012, https://news.harvard.edu/gazette/story/2012/04/berries-keep-your-brain-sharp.

4. E. Devore, J.H. Kang, M. Breteler et al., "Dietary Intakes of Berries and Flavonoids in Relation to Cognitive Decline," *Annals of Neurology* 72, no.1 (2012): 135–143, doi:10.1002/ana.23594.

5. Michael Greger, "Berries vs. Pesticides in Parkinson's Disease," Nutrition Facts, last modified July 13, 2016, https://nutritionfacts.org/video/berries-vs-pesticides-in-parkinsons-disease.

6. P. Pan, Y. Huang, K. Oshima et al., "An Immunological Perspective for Preventing Cancer with Berries," *Journal of Berry Research* 8, no. 3 (January 2018): 163–175, https://content.iospress.com/articles/journal-of-berry-research/jbr180305.

7. F. Aquil, J. Jeyabalan, H. Kauser et al., "Lung Cancer Inhibitory Activity of Dietary Berries and Berry Polyphenolics," *Journal of Berry Research* 6, no. 2 (January 2016): 105–114, https://content.iospress.com/articles/journal-of-berry-research/jbr120.

8. Rani Polak, Edward M. Phillips, and Amy Campbell, "Legumes: Health Benefits and Culinary Approaches to Increase Intake," *Clinical Diabetes* 33, no. 4 (October 2015): 198–205, https://doi.org/10.2337/diaclin.33.4.198.

9. J, Docherty, H. McEwen, T. Sweet et al., "Resveratrol Inhibition of Propionibacterium Acnes," *The Journal of Antimicrobial Chemotherapy* 59, no. 6 (2007): 1182–1184, doi:10.1093/jac/dkm099.

Chapter 5

1. Maria Webster, "The Importance of Sulphur in Your Garden," Family Handyman, last modified November 29, 2022, https://www.familyhandyman.com/article/garden-soil-sulfur.

2. Seema Yadav et al., "Antimicrobial Activity of Fresh Garlic Juice: An In vitro Study.," *Ayu* 36, no. 2 (2015): 203–207, doi:10.410%0974-8520.175548.

3. E. Elnima et al., "The Antimicrobial Activity of Garlic and Onion Extracts.," *Die Pharmazie* 38, no. 11 (1983): 747–748, https://pubmed.ncbi.nlm.nih.gov/6669596/.

4. Taiichiro Seki and Takashi Hosono, "Prevention of Cardiovascular Diseases by Garlic-Derived Sulphur Compounds," *Journal of Nutritional Science and Vitaminology* 61 (2015): S83–S85, https://www.jstage.jst.go.jp/article/jnsv/61/Supplement/61_S83/_pdf/-char/en.

5. Zahra Bahadoran et al., "Allium Vegetable Intakes and the Incidence of Cardiovascular Disease, Hypertension, Chronic Kidney Disease, and Type 2 Diabetes in Adults," *Journal of Hypertension* 35, no. 9 (September 2017): 1909–1916, doi: 10.1097/HJH.0000000000001356.

6. Mahshad Sarvizadeh et al., "Allicin and Digestive System Cancers: From Chemical Structure to Its Therapeutic Opportunities," *Frontiers in Oncology* 11 (April 2021), doi:10.3389/fonc.2021.650256.

7. Ocean Robbins, "Amazing Alliums—Why These Disease Fighting Veggies Are Worth Eating Every Day," Food Revolution Network, last modified July 23, 2021, https://foodrevolution.org/blog/allium-vegetables.

8. Ardini Pangastuti, Sri Endah Indriwati, and Mohamad Amin, "Investigation of the Anti-aging Properties of Allicin from *Allium sativum* L Bulb Extracts by a Reverse Docking Approach," *Tropical Journal of Pharmaceutical Research* 17, no. 4 (2018), https://www.researchgate.net/publication/325066943_Investigation_of_the_anti-aging_properties_of_allicin_from_Allium_sativum_L_bulb_extracts_by_a_reverse_docking_approach.

9. J. Ban, J. Oh, T. Kim et al., "Anti-inflammatory and Arthritic Effects of Thiacremonone, a Novel Sulfur Compound Isolated from Garlic via Inhibition of NF-κB," *Arthritis Research & Therapy* 11, no. R145 (2009), https://doi.org/10.1186/ar2819.

10. "Onions Can Help Prevent Inflammation," Arthritis Foundation, last modified June 1, 2022, http://blog.arthritis.org/living-with-arthritis/onions-prevent-inflammation-arthritis-diet.

11. "Onion Myths and FAQs," National Onion Association, accessed January 24, 2023, https://www.onions-usa.org/tips-onion-myths-faqs/faqs.

Chapter 6

1. Cho et al., "Antioxidant and Anti-Inflammatory Activities in Relation to the Flavonoids Composition of Pepper (*Capsicum annuum* L.)," *Antioxidants* 9, no.10 (2020):986, https://doi.org/10.3390/antiox9100986.

2. Sarah Rautio, "Increase Intake of Fresh Herbs for Everyday Health," MSU Extension, last modified February 17, 2017, https://www.canr.msu.edu/news/increase_intake_of_fresh_herbs_for_everyday_health.

3. Ocean Robbins, "How Curcumin Can Help You Hack Your Genes and Avoid Disease," Food Revolution Network, last modified January 23, 2020, https://foodrevolution.org/blog/health-benefits-of-curcumin.

4. Michael Greger, "Peppermint Oil for Irritable Bowel Syndrome," Nutrition Facts, last modified July 10, 2015, https://nutritionfacts.org/video/peppermint-oil-for-irritable-bowel-syndrome/.

5. Ocean Robbins, "Ginger Benefits and Side Effects," Food Revolution Network, April 22, 2020, https://foodrevolution.org/blog/ginger-benefits-and-side-effects/.

6. Krishnapura Srinivasan, "Cumin (*Cuminum cyminum*) and Black Cumin (*Nigella sativa*) Seeds: Traditional Uses, Chemical Constituents, and Nutraceutical Effects," *Food Quality and Safety* 2, no. 1 (March 2018): 1–16, https://doi.org/10.1093/fqsafe/fyx031.

7. G. J. Kaur and D. S. Arora, "Antibacterial and Phytochemical Screening of *Anethum graveolens, Foeniculum vulgare* and *Trachyspermum ammi*," *BMC Complementary and Alternative Medicine* 9, no. 30 (2009), https://doi.org/10.118%1472-6882-9-30.

8. Shyamapada Mandal and Manisha Mandal, "Coriander (Coriandrum sativum L.) Essential Oil: Chemistry and Biological Activity, *Asian Pacific Journal of Tropical Biomedicine* 5, no. 6, (2015): 421-428, https://www.sciencedirect.com/science/article/pii/S2221169115000647.

9. Ocean Robbins, "Fresh vs. Dried: A Guide to Herbs and Spices," Food Revolution Network.

10. Lindsay Oberst, "How to Stay Healthy and Fight Cancer with Parsley," Food Revolution Network, last modified December 16, 2015, https://foodrevolution.org/blog/parsley-cancer-health.

11. Ocean Robbins, "Fresh vs. Dried: A Guide to Herbs and Spices," Food Revolution Network, last modified November 11, 2021, https://foodrevolution.org/blog/cooking-with-herbs-and-spices-fresh-vs-dried/.

12. Ocean Robbins, "What Is Cumin, and Should You Eat It for Your Health," Food Revolution Network, last modified January 31, 2020, https://foodrevolution.org/blog/health-benefits-of-cumin.

13. Ocean Robbins, "Ginger Benefits and Side Effects," Food Revolution Network.

14. Cho et al., "Antioxidant and Anti-Inflammatory Activities in Relation to the Flavonoids Composition of Pepper (*Capsicum annuum* L.)." 986.

15. Ocean Robbins, "Ginger Benefits and Side Effects," Food Revolution Network.

16. Kuptniratsaikul et al., "Efficacy and Safety of Curcuma domestica Extracts Compared with Ibuprofen in Patients with Knee Osteoarthritis: a Multicenter Study," *Clinical Interventions in Aging* 9 (March 2014): 451–458, doi:10.2147/CIA.S58535.

Chapter 7

1. Aaron Hutcherson, "A Guide to Sweet Potato Varieties," *The Washington Post*, https://www.washingtonpost.com/food/2021/09/24/sweet-potatoes-guide/.

2. "New research suggests sweet potatoes did not originate in the Americas", Indiana University News, last modified May 21, 2018, https://news.iu.edu/live/news/25018-new-research-suggests-sweet-potatoes-did-not

3. Lindeberg et al., "Cardiovascular Risk Factors in a Melanesian Population Apparently Free from Stroke and Ischaemic Heart Disease: the Kitava Study.," *Journal of Internal Medicine* 236, no. 3 (1994): 331-340, doi:10.1111/j.1365-2796.1994.tb00804.x.

4. Daniel J. DeNoon, "Death Stalks Smokers in Beta-Carotene Study," WebMD, November 30, 2004, https://www.webmd.com/smoking-cessation/news/20041130/death-stalks-smokers-in-beta-carotene-study.

5. Cheow Peng Ooi and Seng Cheong Loke, "Sweet Potato for Type 2 Diabetes Mellitus." *The Cochrane Database of Systematic Reviews* 2013, no. 9 (September 2013), doi:10.100²⁄₁₄₆₅₁₈₅₈.CD009128.pub3.

6. Kendra Cherry, "What Is Acetylcholine?" Verywellmind, last modified September 9, 2022, https://www.verywellmind.com/what-is-acetylcholine-2794810.

7. Priyanka Runwal, "Sweet Potato Sends Secret Signals," *Scientific American,* last modified January 24, 2020, https://www.scientificamerican.com/article/sweet-potato-sends-secret-signals/.

Chapter 8

1. Ruth Schuster, "Archaeologists Find 780,000-Year-Old Remains of Prehistoric Man's Meal," *Haaretz*, last modified December 5, 2016, https://www.haaretz.com/archaeology/2016-12-05/ty-article-magazine/780-000-year-old-remains-of-plant-diet-found-in-israel/0000017f-f87e-d887-a7ff-f8fe05f00000.

2. "Healthy Foods High in Selenium," WebMD, last modified November 23, 2022, https://www.webmd.com/diet/foods-high-in-selenium.

3. Ying Bao, "Association of Nut Consumption with Total and Cause-Specific Mortality," *New England Journal of Medicine* 369, no. 21 (November 2013): 2001–2011, https://www.nejm.org/doi/full/10.1056/NEJMoa1307352.

4. Emily Esfahani Smith, "The Lovely Hill: Where People Live Longer and Happier," *The Atlantic*, last modified February 4, 2013, https://www.theatlantic.com/health/archive/2013/02/the-lovely-hill-where-people-live-longer-and-happier/272798.

5. "Nuts and Your Heart: Eating Nuts for Heart Health," Mayo Clinic, last modified August 2, 2022, https://www.mayoclinic.org/diseases-conditions/heart-disease/in-depth/nuts/art-20046635.

6. Mohammadifard et al., "Longitudinal Association of Nut Consumption and the Risk of Cardiovascular Events: A Prospective Cohort Study in the Eastern Mediterranean Region," *Frontiers in Nutrition* 7 no. 610467 (January 2021), doi:10.3389/fnut.2020.610467.

7. Ocean Robbins, "You Won't Believe How Healthy Nuts Are For You," Food Revolution Network, last modified July 29, 2021, https://foodrevolution.org/blog/nuts-health.

8. Edel et al., "Dietary Flaxseed Independently Lowers Circulating Cholesterol and Lowers It Beyond the Effects of Cholesterol-lowering Medications Alone in Patients with Peripheral Artery Disease," *The Journal of Nutrition* 145, no. 4 (2015): 749–757,.https://pubmed.ncbi.nlm.nih.gov/25694068.

9. Kailash Prasad and Ashok Jadhav. "Prevention and Treatment of Atherosclerosis with Flaxseed-derived Compound Secoisolariciresinol Diglucoside." *Current Pharmaceutical Design* 22, no. 2 (2016): 214-220, doi:10.217⁴⁄1381612822666151112151130.

10. Ocean Robbins, "All About Hemp Seeds—A Nutritionally Dense Superfood," Food Revolution Network, June 18, 2020, https://foodrevolution.org/blog/hemp-seeds.

11.   Toscano et al., "Chia Flour Supplementation Reduces Blood Pressure in Hypertensive Subjects," *Plant Foods for Human Nutrition* 69, no. 4 (2014): 392–398, doi:10.1007/s11130-014-0452-7.

12.   Sánchez-González et al., "Walnut Polyphenol Metabolites, Urolithins A and B, Inhibit the Expression of the Prostate-specific Antigen and the Androgen Receptor in Prostate Cancer Cells," *Food & Function* 11 (2014): 2922–2930, https://pubs.rsc.org/en/content/articlelanding/2014/fo/c4fo00542b#!divAbstract.

13.   Sara Bondell, "Eating Walnuts May Help Breast Cancer Patients," Endeavor, last modified April 1, 2019, https://moffitt.org/endeavor/archive/eating-walnuts-may-help-breast-cancer-patients.

14.   Ocean Robbins, "Are Flaxseeds Good For You?—And the Best Way to Eat Them," Food Revolution Network, last modified August 13, 2021, https://foodrevolution.org/blog/is-flaxseed-good-for-you.

15.   Deshpande et al., "Alpha-linolenic Acid Regulates the Growth of Breast and Cervical Cancer Cell Lines through Regulation of NO Release and Induction of Lipid Peroxidation," *Journal of Molecular Biology* (February 2013), http://www.jmolbiochem.com/index.php/JmolBiochem/article/view/52.

16.   Seema Gulati, Anoop Misra, and Ravindra M. Pandey, "Effect of Almond Supplementation on Glycemia and Cardiovascular Risk Factors in Asian Indians in North India with Type 2 Diabetes Mellitus: A 24–Week Study," *Metabolic Syndrome and Related Disorders* 15, no. 2 (2017): 98–105, https://www.ncbi.nlm.nih.gov/pmc/articles/PMC5333560.

17.   Arab et al., "Association Between Walnut Consumption and Diabetes Risk in NHANES," *Diabetes Metabolism Research and Reviews* 34, no. 7 (October 2018), https://onlinelibrary.wiley.com/doi/full/10.1002/dmrr.3031.

18.   Ho et al., "Effect of Whole and Ground Salba Seeds (Salvia Hispanica L.) on Postprandial glycemia in Healthy Volunteers: a Randomized Controlled, Dose-response Trial," *European Journal of Clinical Nutrition* 67, no. 7 (2013): 786–788, doi:10.1038/ejcn.2013.103.

19.   "Worldwide Revenue of Pfizer's Viagra from 2003 to 2017 (in Million U.S. Dollars)," Statistica, February 2018.

20.   Tsai et al., "A Prospective Cohort Study of Nut Consumption and the Risk of Gallstone Disease in Men," *American Journal of Epidemiology* 160, no. 10 (2004): 961–968, doi:10.1093/aje/kwh302.

21.   Aldemir et al., "Pistachio Diet Improves Erectile Function Parameters and Serum Lipid Profiles in Patients with Erectile Dysfunction," *International Journal of Impotence* Research 23 (2011): 32–38, https://doi.org/10.1038/ijir.2010.33.

Chapter 9

1.   "The Discovery of Coffee: The Legend of Kaldi," Waycap Capsules and Coffee, last modified June 19, 2018, https://www.compatible-capsules.com/coffee-culture/discovery-of-coffee-legend-of-kaldi/.

2.   "Legend of Teas," Dethlefsen and Balk, last accessed January 24, 2023, https://www.dethlefsen-balk.de/ENU/10730/Legende_vom_Tee.html.

3.   "Types of Coffee Beans and What Sets Them Apart," District Roasters, last modified March 13, 2019, https://districtroasters.com/blogs/news/types-of-coffee-beans.

4.   Ocean Robbins, "Is Coffee Good for You or Bad for You? Find Out the Truth!" Food Revolution Network, last modified January 20, 2023, https://foodrevolution.org/blog/coffee-health/.

5.   Lopez-Garcia et al., "Coffee Consumption and Risk of Stroke in Women," *Circulation* 119, no. 8 (2009): 1116–1123, doi:10.1161/CIRCULATIONAHA.108.826164.

6.   Susanna Larsson, Jarmo Vitarmo, and Alicja Wolk, "Coffee Consumption and Risk of Stroke in Women," *Stroke* 42, no. 4 (2011): 908–912, doi:10.1161/STROKEAHA.110.603787.

7.   "Coffee," The Nutrition Source, accessed January 24, 2023, https://www.hsph.harvard.edu/nutritionsource/food-features/coffee.

8.   Ocean Robbins, "Tea Health Benefits," Food Revolution Network, last modified May 4, 2020, https://foodrevolution.org/blog/tea-health-benefits.

9. Grassi et al., "Black Tea Consumption Dose-dependently Improves Flow-mediated Dilation in Healthy Males," *Journal of Hypertension* 27, no. 4 (April 2009): 774–781, DOI: 10.1097/HJH.0b013e328326066c.

10. Zheng et al., "Green Tea Intake Lowers Fasting Serum Total and LDL Cholesterol in Adults: a Meta-analysis of 14 Randomized Controlled Trials," *The American Journal of Clinical Nutrition* 94, no. 2 (2011): 601–610, doi:10.3945/ajcn.110.010926.

11. Kuriyama et al., "Green Tea Consumption and Mortality Due to Cardiovascular Disease, Cancer, and All Causes in Japan: The Ohsaki Study," *Journal of the American Medical Association* 296, no. 10 (September 2006): 1255–1265, doi:10.1001/jama.296.10.1255.

12. Ocean Robbins, "What to Eat and Drink for Better Sleep," Food Revolution Network, last modified December 1, 2021, https://foodrevolution.org/blog/food-and-drinks-for-better-sleep.

13. Ocean Robbins, "5 Science-Backed Reasons to Drink Matcha Tea," Food Revolution Network, last modified November 2, 2018, https://foodrevolution.org/blog/matcha-tea-benefits.

14. Büşra Açıkalın and Nevin Sanlier," Coffee and Its Effects on the Immune System," *Trends in Food Science & Technology* 114 (2021): 625–632, https://doi.org/10.1016/j.tifs.2021.06.023.6

15. Benedette Cuffari, "How Does Coffee Affect the Immune System," News Medical, last modified September 8, 2022, https://www.news-medical.net/health/How-Does-Coffee-Affect-the-Immune-System.aspx.

16. Fujiki et al., "Cancer Prevention with Green Tea and Its Principal Constituent, EGCG: from Early Investigations to Current Focus on Human Cancer Stem Cells," *Molecules and Cells* 41, no. 2 (2018): 73–82, doi:10.14348/molcells.2018.2227.

17. Lindsay Oberst, "The Surprising Inflammation and Aging Benefits of Caffeine," Food Revolution Network, last modified July 30, 2021, https://foodrevolution.org/blog/food-and-health/caffeine-coffee-tea-inflammation-anti-aging.

18. Elizabeth Mendes, "Coffee and Cancer: What the Research Really Shows," American Cancer Society, last modified April 3, 2018, https://www.cancer.org/latest-news/coffee-and-cancer-what-the-research-really-shows.html.

19. Eskelinen et al., "Midlife Coffee and Tea Drinking and the Risk of Late-life Dementia: a Population-based CAIDE Study," *Journal of Alzheimer's Disease* 16, no. 1 (2009): 85–91, doi:10.3233/JAD-2009-0920.

20. Hu et al., "Coffee and Tea Consumption and the Risk of Parkinson's Disease," *Movement Disorders* 22, no. 15 (2007): 2242–2248, doi:10.1002/mds.21706.

21. Pervin et al., "Beneficial Effects of Green Tea Catechins on Neurodegenerative Diseases," *Molecules* 23, no. 6 (May 2018): 1297, doi:10.3390/molecules23061297.

22. Torquati et al., "A Daily Cup of Tea or Coffee May Keep You Moving: Association between Tea and Coffee Consumption and Physical Activity," *International Journal of Environmental Research and Public Health* 15, no. 9 (2018):1812, https://doi.org/10.3390/ijerph15091812.

23. Ales Pospisil, "The Ultimate Guide to Homemade Cold Brew Coffee," European Coffee Trip, last modified July 15, 2020, https://europeancoffeetrip.com/how-to-make-cold-brew-coffee/.

24. "The Six Immutable Laws of Tea Storage," Tea Epicure, accessed January 24, 2023, https://teaepicure.com/how-to-store-tea/.

25. "Lipton Lemon Iced Tea," Fatsecret, accessed January 24, 2023, https://www.fatsecret.com/calories-nutrition/lipton/lemon-iced-tea.

APPENDIX

SUPERFOOD NUTRIENTS Use this guide as a quick reference to find the superfoods and their key nutrients, as well as get inspiration for how to use them in your next meal. As you can see, well-rounded plant-based nutrition doesn't have to come from exotic foods!

SUPERFOOD	KEY NUTRIENTS	HOW TO USE
Leafy Greens	carotenoids • chlorophyll B vitamins • vitamin A • vitamin E vitamin K • calcium iron • magnesium	salads • stir-fries steamed/sautéed • sides soups/stews casseroles • smoothies • dips
Mushrooms	ergothioneine • glutathione B vitamins • vitamin D (when they're exposed to the sun while growing) selenium • potassium copper • dietary fibers: beta-glucans and chitin	casseroles • classic pizza topping soups • stews • stir-fries sandwiches/wraps • veggie burgers meat replacement
Legumes	protein • fiber • resistant starch phytochemicals • flavonoids B vitamins (especially folate) • iron calcium • zinc magnesium	salads • salad topping stir-fries • soups/stews casseroles • dips/sauces pasta • grain bowls desserts • veggie burger base
Berries	anthocyanins • polyphenols fiber • vitamin C manganese • vitamin K1	on their own • fruit salad fruit compote • in baked dessert popsicles • dessert topping smoothies • smoothie bowls dressings/sauces
Alliums	sulfurs • soluble fibers: fructans and inulin • B vitamins (especially folate) vitamin C • potassium • selenium manganese	sauces • soups/stews stir-fries • scrambles pasta dishes • grain bowls salads • mains
Sweet Potatoes	fiber • resistant starch vitamin C • carotenoids beta-carotene (which gives the orange ones their color) B vitamins manganese • magnesium • copper	baked with toppings • seasonal side dishes chilis/stews • casseroles grain bowls • hashes desserts (brownies and sweet potato pies)
Nuts and Seeds	protein • fiber • healthy fats tocopherols (Vitamin E) phytosterols magnesium • iron • phosphorus calcium • zinc	raw or roasted on their own nut-based flour/meal • nut butter • trail mix • granola • salad toppers • stir-fries toppers • desserts • dressings • dips spreads • nut and seed milks smoothies • nut cheeses
Herbs and Spices (nutrients vary depending on the herbs and spices)	vitamin C • carotenoids • flavonoids vitamins A • vitamin K • iron magnesium • calcium • manganese omega-3 and -6 fatty acids	sweet herbs/spices: desserts sauces • hot drinks • savory herbs/spice: soups/stews • mains casseroles • salads dressings/sauces grain bowls • sides
Tea and Coffee	Coffee: hydrocinnamic acids polyphenols Green tea: catechins/EGCG L-theanine Black tea: polyphenols	smoothies • desserts/baked goods warm cup on its own with a splash of plant milk

THE WONDERFUL WORLD OF MUSHROOMS

MUSHROOM TYPE	BENEFITS
White (button, portobello, and cremini)	Support healthy immune function Rich in antioxidants • Antiaging Anticancer • Support healthy brain function and cognition Heart healthy Support healthy digestion
Shiitake	Support healthy immune function Heart healthy • Lower cholesterol Maintain healthy blood pressure Rich in antioxidants
Enoki	Support healthy immune function Anticancer • Heart healthy Support healthy brain function and cognition Rich in antioxidants
Lion's Mane	Support healthy immune function Focus, mental clarity, and mood Reduce anxiety symptoms • Anti-inflammatory Rich in antioxidants
Turkey Tail	Support healthy immune function Anticancer • Rich in antioxidants
Hen of the Woods (maitake)	Support healthy immune function Anticancer • Lower cholesterol Blood sugar control • Anti-inflammatory
Beech (shimeji)	Support healthy immune function Rich in antioxidants • Anti-inflammatory Antimicrobial • Lower cholesterol Heart healthy
Chanterelle	Support healthy immune function Rich in antioxidants Support bone health
Porcini	Support healthy immune function Anti-inflammatory • Antiviral/antibacterial Support healthy digestion • Reduce risk of cardiovascular disease • Rich in antioxidants
Morel	Supports healthy immune function Anti-tumor • Anti-inflammatory Rich in antioxidants
Oyster	Support healthy immune function Reduce high blood pressure Lower cholesterol • Blood sugar control Heart healthy • Rich in antioxidants
Chaga	Support healthy immune function Reduce oxidative stress • Rich in antioxidants Anti-inflammatory Lower cholesterol • Anticancer Blood sugar control • Antitumor Heart healthy

HOW TO COOK BEANS GUIDE
Beans are not only a great source of protein and fiber, they are also concentrated with plenty of the vitamins and minerals your body needs to thrive. Enjoy experimenting with these wholesome varieties—what you can create in the kitchen is endless!

BEANS (1 CUP DRIED)	WATER	SOAK TIME	COOK TIME	COOKED AMOUNT
Adzuki Beans	2 ½ cups or until completely covered	Hot Soak: 4 hours Quick Soak: 1–2 hours Overnight: 8–12 hours	Stovetop: 3 5–45 minutes Pressure Cooker: 15–20 minutes	3–3 ½ cups
Black Beans	2 ½ cups or until completely covered	Hot Soak: 4 hours Quick Soak: 1–2 hours Overnight: 8–12 hours	Stovetop: 50–60 minutes Pressure Cooker: 8–10 minutes	3–3 ½ cups
Black-Eyed Peas	2 ½ cups or until completely covered	Hot Soak: 4 hours Quick Soak: 1-2 hours Overnight: 8-12 hours	Stovetop: 45–60 minutes Pressure Cooker: 8–10 minutes	3–3 ½ cups
Butter Beans/ Lima Beans	2 ½ cups or until completely covered	Hot Soak: 4 hours Quick Soak: 1–2 hours Overnight: 8–12 hours	Stovetop: 45–60 minutes Pressure Cooker: 12–15 minutes	3–3 ½ cups
Cannellini Beans	2 ½ cups or until completely covered	Hot Soak: 4 hours Quick Soak: 1–2 hours Overnight: 8–12 hours	Stovetop: 90 minutes–2 hours Pressure Cooker: 20–30 minutes	3–3 ½ cups
Fava Beans	2 ½ cups or until completely covered	Hot Soak: 4 hours Quick Soak: 1–2 hours Overnight: 8–12 hours	Stovetop: 50–70 minutes Pressure Cooker: 8–11 minutes	3–3 ½ cups
Edamame (fresh)	2 ½ cups or until completely covered	No soaking required	Stovetop: 5–10 minutes Pressure Cooker: 1–2 minutes	1 cup

Garbanzo Beans/ Chickpeas	2 ½ cups until completely covered	Hot Soak: 4 hours Quick Soak: 1–2 hours Overnight: 8–12 hours	Stovetop: 90 minutes–3 hours Pressure Cooker: 15–20 minutes	3–3 ½ cups
Great Northern Beans	2 ½ cups or until completely covered	Hot Soak: 4 hours Quick Soak: 1–2 hours Overnight: 8–12 hours	Stovetop: 45–60 minutes Pressure Cooker: 12–15 mintues	3–3 ½ cups
Lentils (brown)	2 ½ cups or until completely covered	No soaking required	Stovetop: 30–40 minutes Pressure Cooker: 7–10 minutes	3–3 ½ cups
Lentils (green)	2 ½ cups or until completely covered	No soaking required	Stovetop: 30–40 minutes Pressure Cooker: 7–10 minutes	3–3 ½ cups
Lentils (red)	2 ½ cups or until completely covered	No soaking required	Stovetop: 15–25 minutes Pressure Cooker: 7–8 minutes	3–3 ½ cups (note red lentils cook down to a paste like consistency)
Mung Beans	2 ½ cups or until completely covered	Hot Soak: 4 hours Quick Soak: 1–2 hours Overnight: 8–12 hours	Stovetop: 50–70 minutes Pressure Cooker: 6–8 minutes	3–3 ½ cups
Navy Beans	2 ½ cups or until completely covered	Hot Soak: 4 hours Quick Soak: 1–2 hours Overnight: 8–12 hours	Stovetop: 45–60 minutes Pressure Cooker: 7–10 minutes	3–3 ½ cups

Pinto Beans	2 ½ cups or until completely covered	Hot Soak: 4 hours Quick Soak: 1–2 hours Overnight: 8–12 hours	Stovetop: 60–90 minutes Pressure Cooker: 8–10 minutes	3–3 ½ cups
Red Beans/Small Kidney Bean	2 ½ cups or until completely covered	Hot Soak: 4 hours Quick Soak: 1–2 hours Overnight: 8–12 hours	Stovetop: 70–90 minutes Pressure Cooker: 12–15 minutes	3–3 ½ cups
Soybeans	2 ½ cups or until completely covered	Hot Soak: 4 hours Quick Soak: 1–2 hours Overnight: 8–12 hours	Stovetop: 2 ½–3 hours Pressure Cooker: 15–20 minutes	3–3 ½ cups
Split Peas	2 ½ cups or until completely covered	No soaking required	Stovetop: 35–45 minutes Pressure Cooker: 5–8 minutes	3–3 ½ cups
Whole Peas	2 ½ cups or until completely covered	Hot Soak: 4 hours Quick Soak: 1–2 hours Overnight: 8–12 hours	Stovetop: 45–60 minutes Pressure Cooker: 6–10 minutes	3–3 ½ cups

GENERAL DIRECTIONS

1. Pick through the beans, discarding any discolored or shriveled beans.

2. Rinse the beans well.

3. Soak the beans according to the suggested times and methods above.

4. Place over medium heat; keep water at a gentle simmer to prevent split skins.

5. Beans expand in size as they soak and cook, so it is important to keep an eye on the water-to-bean ratio. Add warm water periodically during the cooking process to keep the beans covered.

6. Stir beans occasionally throughout the cooking process to prevent sticking to the bottom of the pot.

7. Beans take 30 minutes to 2 hours to cook on the stovetop, depending on the variety. You will know the beans are done when they are tender but not mushy.

COOKING METHODS

Depending on how you'd like to cook your beans, most bean varieties (after soaking) cook within 30 minutes to 2 hours. Cooking beans using a pressure cooker helps to reduce the time and takes the guesswork out of knowing when the beans are tender; it gets it perfect every time! The pressure and steam also penetrate the tough exterior of beans, making them easier to digest. If you don't have one, a pot or slow cooker can work well, too.

Tip: Add a bay leaf or a strip of dried kombu (a sea vegetable) when cooking beans. Doing so not only adds flavor, but the kombu can help tenderize the beans and reduce flatulence during digestion. Kombu contains alpha-galactosidase, which helps break down the oligosaccharides in beans that are responsible for their gastrointestinal irritation. You can also add spices, such as fennel, cumin, caraway, ginger, epazote, asafoetida, and turmeric to help make beans more digestible.

WHY PRE-SOAK YOUR BEANS BEFORE COOKING?

Soaking beans allows the dried beans to absorb water, which begins to dissolve the antinutrients that cause intestinal discomfort and gas. While beans are soaking they are also expanding in size, which results in faster cooking times. To learn more about the benefits of soaking beans to reduce antinutrients visit our blog post at foodrevolution.org, *What are Antinutrients? And Do You Need To Avoid Them?*

SOAKING METHODS

Hot soak: If you are unable to soak your beans overnight, hot soaking is an easy way to help soften the beans and wash away some of the antinutrients before cooking. Simply add 3 to 4 cups of water to a pot and bring to a boil (4 to 5 minutes). Remove the water from the heat, add your beans, and cover with a tight-fitting lid. Allow the beans to soak for 4 hours. Then drain the water, add fresh water to the beans, and cook using your preferred method of choice.

Quick soak: Quick soaking is the fastest method and it will help to soften the beans and remove some antinutrients, but it is not as effective as other soaking methods. However, lentils (they only need about 20 to 30 minutes) are ideal for this method if antinutrients are a concern. Simply add 2 to 3 cups of water to a pot and bring to a boil (4 to 5 minutes). Remove the water from the heat, add your beans, and cover with a tight-fitting lid. Allow the beans to soak for 1 to 2 hours. Then drain the water, add fresh water to the beans, and cook using your preferred method of choice.

Overnight soak: Overnight soaking is the easiest method and the most effective for removing antinutrients. You can soak your beans anywhere from 8 to 24 hours. In a large container, add 4 cups of water and cover. If you extend the soaking time past 12 hours, discard the original soaking liquid, rinse, and resoak in fresh water about 2 to 3 times per day. Then drain the water, add fresh water to the beans, and cook using your preferred method of choice.

BATCH COOKING

Cook beans in large batches so you have them ready to go for the week or freeze them for weeks to come. Batch cooking can save you time in the kitchen. Cooked beans keep 3 to 4 days in the refrigerator and take a minimal amount of time to reheat. Use beans in salads and grain bowls, as the base for plant burgers, or toss them in your favorite soups or stews. You can also store cooked beans in the freezer for a few months, portioning them in individual containers and using them as you need. After you cook your batched beans, spread them out on a parchment-lined baking sheet so that they cool completely before storing and the beans do not clump together. Freeze the cooled beans, then move them to an airtight container for proper freezer storage.

GARLIC VARIETIES Garlic is most commonly grown in white, purple, and pink varieties.

Hardneck (*Allium sativum var ophioscorodon*) In the hardneck family, there are eight subtypes of garlic: Purple Stripe, Marbled Purple Stripe, Asiatic, Glazed Purple Stripe, Creole, Turban, Rocambole, and Porcelain	Softneck (*Allium sativum var. sativum*) In the softneck family, there are three subtypes of garlic: Artichoke, Middle Eastern and Silverskin
Asian Tempest (Seoul Sister): Asiatic	**Acropolis Greek:** Artichoke
Bogatyr: Marbled Purple Stripe	**Corsican Red:** Artichoke
Brown Tempest: Glazed Purple Stripe	**Inchelium Red:** Artichoke
Chesnok Red: Purple Stripe	**Kettle River Giant:** Artichoke
Danube Rose: Porcelain	**Loz Italian:** Artichoke
German Extra Hardy: Porcelain	**Nootka Rose:** Artichoke
German Porcelain: Porcelain	**Printanor:** Artichoke
German Red: Rocambole	**Red Toch (Tochiliavir):** Artichoke
Italian Purple: Rocambole	**Rose du Lautrec:** Silverskin
Killarney Red: Rocambole	**Rose du Var:** Silverskin
Korean Red: Purple Stripe	**RojodelPaisBaza:** Creole/Silverskin (dependant on growing conditions)
Morasol: Purple Stripe	**Shantung Purple:** Softneck
Music: Porcelain	**Thermadrome:** Artichoke
RojodelPaisBaza: Creole	**Transylvanian:** Artichoke
Sandpoint Rocambole: Rocambole	
Siberian: Marbled Purple Stripe	
Spanish Roja: Rocambole	
Stull: Porcelain	
Vekak Czech: Glazed Purple Stripe	
Vostani: Porcelain	

ONION VARIETIES AND HOW TO USE THEM

TYPE	FLAVOR	CULINARY USE
Chives	Delicate	An herby garnish to bakes/casseroles • dips potatoes • soups
Cipollini (Italian pearl onion)	Sweet, buttery when cooked	grilled • roasted caramelized/glazed stewed • creamed
Leeks	Earthly, pungent, sweet	greens: used as flavor agent to homemade vegetable stock whites: bakes/casseroles dressings • pasta sautés • soups/stews
Pearl onion (cocktail onions)	Delicate, sweet	creamed • glazed/caramelized • pickled roasted • stewed
Ramps (North American native spring onion)	Garlicky, pungent, mildly sweet	whites and greens/purples: quick breads raw as a garnish • stir-fries rice dishes • dips • salads soups noodles/pasta
Red onion	Bright, pungent, sharp	garnish on top of stews pickled • salads sandwiches/wraps
Sweet onion (Vidalia onion, Maui onion)	Mild, sweet	caramelized • onion rings soups/stews • sautés
Shallots	Pungent, garlicky, mildly sweet	raw uses: marinades salads • vinaigrettes cooked uses: bakes/casseroles soups/stews • sauces • sautés quiches
Scallions (green onions/spring onions)	Bright, fresh, savory	whites and greens: sautés • quick breads raw as a garnish: dips dressings • noodles/pasta rice dishes • salads soups/stews • stir-fries
White onion	Fresh, slightly tangy, savory	raw as a garnish: guacamole salsa/pico de gallo tacos
Yellow globe onion (Spanish onion)	Not too sweet and not too sharp	bakes/casseroles caramelized • curries mirepoix, soffritto, holy trinity stir-fries • sauces soups/stews • rice dishes

EVERYDAY HERBS & SPICES Culinary herbs and spices unlock a world of fresh, vibrant, and tantalizing flavors to plant-based meals. Reference these herbs and spices in each cuisine category to inspire your next culinary creation!

JAPANESE	MEXICAN	ITALIAN	THAI	MOROCCAN	GREEK	INDIAN
Basil	Chili	Basil	Sweet Thai Basil	Cardamom	Cilantro	Black Pepper
Cardamon	Cilantro	Garlic	Cilantro	Clove	Cinnamon	Cardamom
Chili	Cinnamon	Marjoram	Chili	Chive	Chili	Chili
Garlic	Coriander	Onion	Cumin	Cilantro	Dill	Cinnamon
Ginger	Cumin	Oregano	Curry	Cinnamon	Fenugreek	Clove
Miso	Garlic	Parsley	Lime	Coriander	Garlic	Cumin
Scallion	Onion	Rosemary	Mint	Cumin	Marjoram	Curry
Sesame	Paprika (sweet and smoked)	Sage	Sesame	Fenugreek	Mint	Garam masala
	Saffron	Thyme	Turmeric	Garlic	Onion	Garlic
		White Pepper	Tamarind	Mint	Oregano	Ginger
				Ginger	Parsley	Fennel seed
				Saffron	Sumac	Mint
					Thyme	Onion
						Tamarind
						Turmeric

SWEET POTATO VARIETIES Look for a few of these delicious sweet potato varieties during your next farmer's market or co-op visit!

Covington	**Skin:** Rosy • **Flesh:** Deep orange
Darby	**Skin:** Deep red • **Flesh:** Deep orange
Jewel	**Skin:** Coppery • **Flesh:** Bright orange
Bunch Porto-Rico	**Skin:** Yellow orange • **Flesh:** Yellow orange
Excel	**Skin:** Orange tan • **Flesh:** Coppery orange
Evangeline	**Skin:** Rosy • **Flesh:** Deep orange
Heartogold	Skin: Tan • **Flesh:** Deep orange
Red garnet	**Skin:** Reddish purple • **Flesh:** Orange
Vardaman	**Skin:** Pale orange • **Flesh:** Reddish orange
Murasaki	**Skin:** Reddish purple • **Flesh:** White
Gloden Slipper (Heirloom)	**Skin:** Pale orange • **Flesh:** Pale orange
Carolina Ruby	**Skin:** Deep reddish-purple • **Flesh:** Dark orange
O'Henry	**Skin:** Creamy white • **Flesh:** White
Bienville	**Skin:** Pale rose • **Flesh:** Dark orange
Envy	**Skin:** Pale orange • **Flesh:** Pale orange

(CONTINUED)

Sumor	**Skin:** Creamy tan • **Flesh:** Tan to yellow
Hayman (Heirloom)	**Skin:** Creamy • **Flesh:** Creamy
Jubilee	**Skin:** Creamy • **Flesh:** Creamy
Nugget	**Skin:** Light pink • **Flesh:** Pale orange
Carolina Bunch	**Skin:** Pale coppery orange **Flesh:** Carrot colored
Centennial	**Skin:** Coppery • **Flesh:** Pale orange
Bugs Bunny	**Skin:** Pinkish red • **Flesh**: Pale orange
California Gold	**Skin:** Pale orange • **Flesh:** Orange
Georgia Jet	**Skin:** Reddish purple • **Flesh:** Deep orange

HEALTHY FATS BY THE NUT OR SEED

Monounsaturated Fat: From a health perspective, this type of fat may help to reduce cholesterol, lower your risk of cardiovascular disease, reduce inflammation and maintain the integrity of your body's cells, as they are an essential part of the cell's membranes and are necessary for the absorption of fat-soluble vitamins (vitamins A, E, K, and D).

Polyunsaturated Fat: Polyunsaturated fat is broken down into two main types: omega-3 and omega-6 fatty acids that are essential in your diet. These sources of dietary fats support the proper functioning of nerves and the brain, help maintain the integrity of the skin and other tissues, and are necessary for the absorption of fat-soluble vitamins. Maintaining a good balance between the omega-3 and the omega-6 ratio is important for optimal health.

Omega-3 Fatty Acids: Omega-3 fatty acids have three main forms: ALA (alpha-linolenic acid), which is found in plant foods, EPA (eicosapentaenoic acid), and DHA (docosahexaenoic acid), which is found in algae, fish and other seafood. This form of polyunsaturated fat is anti-inflammatory and essential for brain health.

NUTS/SEEDS	TYPE OF HEALTHY FAT AND KEY NUTRIENTS	BENEFITS
Almonds	Monounsaturated fat Polyunsaturated fat Vitamin E Copper Manganese Magnesium Riboflavin (B2) Phosphorus	Reduces cholesterol Lowers blood pressure Reduces oxidative stress/rich in antioxidants Blood glucose control Weight maintenance/weight loss Anti-inflammatory
Brazil Nuts	Monounsaturated fat Polyunsaturated fat Selenium Maganese Magnesium Thiamin (B1) Phosphorus Zinc Vitamin E	Supports thyroid function Anti-inflammatory Reduces risk of cardiovascular disease Lowers cholesterol levels Supports brain health
Cashew nuts	Monounsaturated fat and Polyunsaturated fat Copper Magnesium Iron Manganese Zinc Selenium	Lowers triglycerides Lowers blood pressure Reduces risk of cardiovascular disease Blood glucose control Weight maintenance/weight loss
Chia seeds	Polyunsaturated fat Monounsaturated fat Omega 3-fatty acids Calcium Iron Magnesium Phosphorus Potassium Zinc Copper Folate Manganese Vitamin C Vitamin E High in fiber	Supports brain health Supports bone health Anti-inflammatory Blood glucose control Reduces risk of cardiovascular disease Supports healthy skin

NUTS/SEEDS	TYPE OF HEALTHY FAT AND KEY NUTRIENTS	BENEFITS
Flaxseeds	Omega 3 fatty acids Polyunsaturated fat Monounsaturated fat Thamin (B1) Pyriodxine (B6) Folate Calcium Copper Iron Mangesium Managnese Phosphorus Selenium Zinc	Reduces oxidative stress/rich in antioxidants Lowers cholesterol Lowers blood pressure Reduces risk of cardiovascular disease Supports mood and brain health Anti-inflammatory Blood glucose control Supports healthy skin
Hemp seeds	Polyunsaturated fat Omega 3-fatty acids Monounsaturated fat Vitamin A (beta-carotene) Thiamin (B1) Niacin (B3) Vitamin B6 Folate Vitamin C Vitamin E Calcium Iron Magnesium Manganese Phosphorus Potassium Zinc High in fiber	Reduces oxidative stress/rich in antioxidants Supports brain health Lowers cholesterol Lowers blood pressure Reduces risk of cardiovascular disease Supports healthy skin

NUTS/SEEDS	TYPE OF HEALTHY FAT AND KEY NUTRIENTS	BENEFITS
Peanuts	Monounsaturated fat Polyunsaturated fat Niacin (B3) Pantothenic acid (B5) Folate Calcium Iron Magnesium Phosphorus Potassium Selenium Zinc High in fiber CoQ-10	Anti-inflammatory Blood sugar control Reduces risk of metabolic syndrome Reduces risk of cardiovascular disease Supports a healthy immune system Hormone regulation Reduces oxidative stress/rich in antioxidants Supports a healthy nervous system Reduces the risk of developing gallstones Protective against Alzheimer's and age-related cognitive decline Supports brain health
Pumpkin seeds	Polyunsaturated fat Monounsaturated fat Riboflavin (B2) Niacin (B3) Folate Vitamin E Vitamin K Choline Calcium Iron Magnesium Phosphorus Potassium Selenium Zinc Copper High in fiber	Improves bladder function Support brain health Supports eye health Antimicrobial/antibacterial Reduces oxidative stress/rich in antioxidants Blood sugar control Supports a healthy immune system Lowers cholesterol Lowers blood pressure Reduces risk of cardiovascular disease

NUTS/SEEDS	TYPE OF HEALTHY FAT AND KEY NUTRIENTS	BENEFITS
Sesame seeds	Polyunsaturated fat Monounsaturated fat Vitamin A (beta carotene) Niacin (B3) Folate Vitamin E Choline Calcium Iron Magnesium Phosphorus Potassium Selenium Zinc	Anti-inflammatory Antiarthritic Lowers cholesterol Reduces oxidative stress/ rich in antioxidants Reduces risk of cardiovascular disease Supports brain health Blood sugar control
Sunflower seeds	Polyunsaturated fat Monounsaturated fat Niacin (B3) Folate Vitamin E Vitamin K Choline Calcium Iron Magnesium Phosphorus Potassium Selenium Zinc	Anti-inflammatory Lowers cholesterol Reduces oxidative stress/ rich in antioxidants Reduces risk of cardiovascular disease Reduces oxidative stress
Walnuts	Polyunsaturated fat Monounsaturated fat Omega-3 fatty acids Copper Maganese Magnesium	Ant-inflammatory Lowers cholesterol Reduces oxidative stress Reduces risk of cardiovascular disease Lowers blood pressure Reduces oxidative stress Supports brain health Supports healthy skin Blood sugar control Supports a healthy gut Blood sugar control Supports male reproductive health

METRIC CONVERSION CHART

Standard Cup	Fine Powder (e.g., flour)	Grain (e.g., rice)	Granular (e.g., sugar)	Liquid Solids (e.g., butter)	Liquid (e.g., milk)
1	140 g	150 g	190 g	200 g	240 ml
¾	105 g	113 g	143 g	150 g	180 ml
⅔	93 g	100 g	125 g	133 g	160 ml
½	70 g	75 g	95 g	100 g	120 ml
⅓	47 g	50 g	63 g	67 g	80 ml
¼	35 g	38 g	48 g	50 g	60 ml
⅛	18 g	19 g	24 g	25 g	30 ml

Useful Equivalents for Cooking/Oven Temperatures

Process	Fahrenheit	Celsius	Gas Mark
Freeze Water	32° F	0° C	
Room Temperature	68° F	20° C	
Boil Water	212° F	100° C	
Bake	325° F	160° C	3
	350° F	180° C	4
	375° F	190° C	5
	400° F	200° C	6
	425° F	220° C	7
	450° F	230° C	8
Broil			Grill

Useful Equivalents for Liquid Ingredients by Volume

¼ tsp				1 ml
½ tsp				2 ml
1 tsp				5 ml
3 tsp	1 tbsp		½ fl oz	15 ml
	2 tbsp	⅓ cup	1 fl oz	30 ml
	4 tbsp	¼ cup	2 fl oz	60 ml
	5 ⅓ tbsp	⅓ cup	3 fl oz	80 ml
	8 tbsp	½ cup	4 fl oz	120 ml
	10 ⅔ tbsp	⅓ cup	5 fl oz	160 ml
	12 tbsp	¾ cup	6 fl oz	180 ml
	16 tbsp	1 cup	8 fl oz	240 ml
	1 pt	2 cups	16 fl oz	480 ml
	1 qt	4 cups	32 fl oz	960 ml
			33 fl oz	1000 ml	1 L

Useful Equivalents for Dry Ingredients by Weight

(To convert ounces to grams, multiply the number of ounces by 30.)

1 oz	⅟₁₆ lb	30 g
4 oz	¼ lb	120 g
8 oz	½ lb	240 g
12 oz	¾ lb	360 g
16 oz	1 lb	480 g

Useful Equivalents for Length

(To convert inches to centimeters, multiply the number of inches by 2.5.)

1 in			2.5 cm	
6 in	½ ft		15 cm	
12 in	1 ft		30 cm	
36 in	3 ft	1 yd	90 cm	
40 in			100 cm	1 m

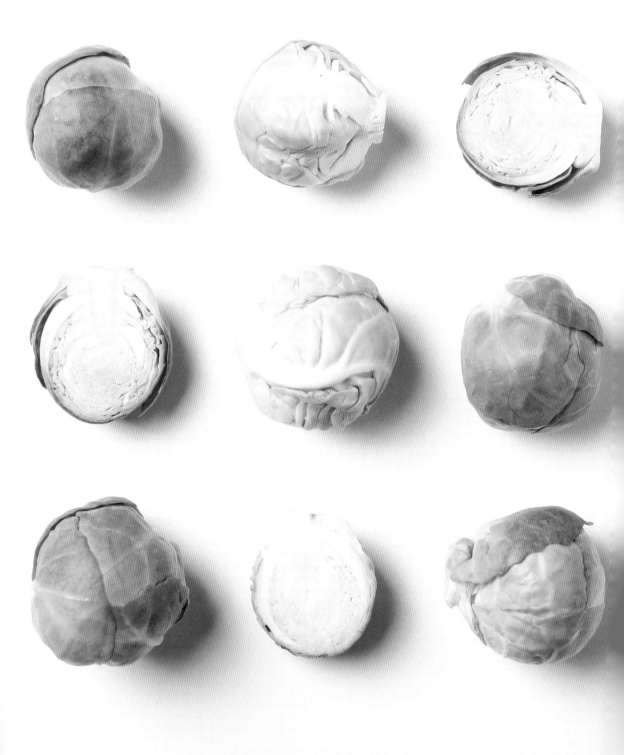

INDEX

ACKNOWLEDGMENTS

Our gratitude and thanks to our partners, Phoenix Robbins and Ricky Russert, and to all of our family members and loved ones who nurture us, support us, share honest feedback, and love us, no matter how obsessed we become with late-night research projects and bizarre culinary creations.

Special thanks to Bobbie Dandrea, recipe tester, editor, and mom.

We are grateful to John Robbins, who has inspired both of us (in very different but truly profound ways), and whose life work led to the launch of Food Revolution Network.

Thank you to Howard Jacobson, whose eloquence and humor have added so much to this book; to AnnMarie Roth, for shepherding this book every step of the way; to Roselynne Mackay, for your creativity and collaborative spirit; to Angela MacNeil, for bringing these recipes to life with your photographic brilliance; to Liana Minassian, for creating the essential framework with which this book was written; to Esther Ender, for your keen proofreading eye; and to the entire team at Food Revolution Network, for your essential support in making this book possible. Working with all of you is a joy and a privilege of the highest magnitude.

Thank you to Reid Tracy, Patty Gift, Lisa Cheng, Monica O'Connor, and the entire editorial and design teams at Hay House, for inspiring this book, believing in us, and bringing this project into the world. We love working with all of you.

And thank you to you, dear reader, for caring about what you eat, and about how it impacts your health and your planet. Together, one bite at a time, we are building healthier lives and a healthier future for life on this planet. Deliciously.

ABOUT THE AUTHORS

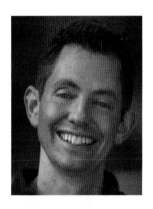

OCEAN ROBBINS is co-founder and CEO of the 750,000+ member Food Revolution Network and author of the best-selling *31-Day Food Revolution*. Ocean founded Youth for Environmental Sanity (YES!) at age 16 and directed it for 20 years. He has spoken at and organized events reaching more than two million people from 65 nations. He has served as adjunct professor for Chapman University and is a recipient of the national Jefferson Award for Outstanding Public Service, the Freedom's Flame Award, the Harmon Wilkinson Award, and many other honors. You can visit him online at **foodrevolution.org**.

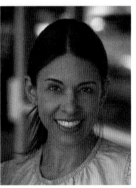

Nichole Dandrea-Russert, MS, RDN, is Food Revolution Network's Lead Dietitian and Recipe Developer. She specializes in women's health, heart disease, and diabetes. She is the author of *The Fiber Effect* and *The Vegan Athlete's Nutrition Handbook*. She lives in Atlanta with her husband and rescue pup, Mariposa. You can visit her online at **www.purelyplanted.com**.

JOIN THE FOOD REVOLUTION

If you've been inspired by the message of this book, please join us in standing for healthy, ethical, and sustainable food for all. You'll gain access to potent resources, a robust global community, and cutting-edge insights to support and deepen your Food Revolution journey. Find out more at **foodrevolution.org/superfoods**.

HAY HOUSE TITLES
OF RELATED INTEREST

YOU CAN HEAL YOUR LIFE, the movie,
starring Louise Hay & Friends
(available as an online streaming video)
www.hayhouse.com/louise-movie

THE SHIFT, the movie,
starring Dr. Wayne W. Dyer
(available as an online streaming video)
www.hayhouse.com/the-shift-movie

***

*BEAT CANCER KITCHEN: Deliciously Simple
Plant-Based Anticancer Recipes,* by Chris Wark

*FOOD BABE KITCHEN: More than 100 Delicious,
Real Food Recipes to Change Your Body and Your Life,* by Vani Hari

*THE FOOD MATTERS COOKBOOK: A Simple Gluten-Free
Guide to Transforming Your Health One Meal at a Time,*
by James Colquhoun & Laurentine ten Bosch

*HEALTHY AT LAST: A Plant-Based Approach to Preventing
and Reversing Diabetes and Other Chronic Illnesses,* by Eric Adams

*THE OFFICIAL BRIGHT LINE EATING COOKBOOK:
Weight Loss Made Simple,* by Susan Peirce Thompson, Ph.D.

All of the above are available at your local bookstore,
or may be ordered by contacting Hay House (see next page).

We hope you enjoyed this Hay House book. If you'd like to receive our online catalog featuring additional information on Hay House books and products, or if you'd like to find out more about the Hay Foundation, please contact:

Hay House LLC, P.O. Box 5100, Carlsbad, CA 92018-5100
(760) 431-7695 or (800) 654-5126
www.hayhouse.com® • www.hayfoundation.org

———

Published in Australia by:
Hay House Australia Publishing Pty Ltd
18/36 Ralph St., Alexandria NSW 2015
Phone: +61 (02) 9669 4299
www.hayhouse.com.au

Published in the United Kingdom by:
Hay House UK Ltd
The Sixth Floor, Watson House,
54 Baker Street, London W1U 7BU
Phone: +44 (0) 203 927 7290
www.hayhouse.co.uk

Published in India by:
Hay House Publishers (India) Pvt Ltd
Muskaan Complex, Plot No. 3,
B-2, Vasant Kunj, New Delhi 110 070
Phone: +91 11 41761620
www.hayhouse.co.in

———

Let Your Soul Grow

Experience life-changing transformation—one video
at a time—with guidance from the world's leading experts.

www.healyourlifeplus.com

MEDITATE.
VISUALIZE.
LEARN.

Get the **Empower You**
Unlimited Audio *Mobile App*

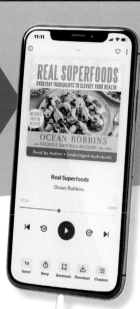

Get unlimited access to the entire Hay House audio library!

You'll get:

- 500+ inspiring and life-changing **audiobooks**

- 200+ ad-free **guided meditations** for sleep, healing, relaxation, spiritual connection, and more

- Hundreds of audios **under 20 minutes** to easily fit into your day

- **Exclusive content** *only* for subscribers

- **New audios** added every week

- No credits, **no limits**

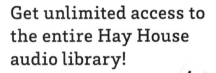

Listen to the audio version of this book for FREE!

 I ADORE this app. I use it almost every day. Such a blessing. – Aya Lucy Rose

Scan me with your phone camera!

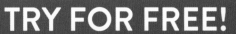

TRY FOR FREE!
Go to: hayhouse.com/listen-free